Aromatherapy, Crystals & Vibrational Healing

Library of Congress Control Number: 2006936141
ISBN # 0-9644198-4-X

First edition, 2006

Cover design by Yavanna Botelho Cook
Cover art by Kendra Grace
Diagrams by Kendra Grace
Botanical illustrations and alchemical symbol
from 15th Century art
Editorial design by Dianna Jacobsen
Editing by Anila Manning

The written material within this book refers to historical and personal data. The author holds no claims regarding the therapeutic uses of essential oils, crystals or other natural elements. This book has the purpose of educating and should not be used as a substitute for traditional medical care.

Nature's Geometry Publications
Post Office Box 656
Laguna Beach, California 92652
Printed in the United States of America

Aromatherapy, Crystals & Vibrational Healing

Kendra Grace

2006
NATURE'S GEOMETRY PUBLICATIONS
LAGUNA BEACH, CALIFORNIA, USA

To Brian

My beloved and life partner,
who has stood behind me and supported everything I ever
wanted to do since my teen years, so I could be free to grow,
evolve and expand. For his amazing transmission from
his zoomed-in vision of the earth, and for his gift of three
magical daughters, Yavanna, Quendi and Natasha.

Acknowledgements

In the course of writing a book, most authors find people
who are torch holders in the dark night of uncertainty,
and who hold our hand crossing the wilderness
where wild beasts may lurk.
For me, with this edition, my warmest thanks go to:

Anada, for that walk across the bridge to the tea house
where we had enlightening conversations and
played word catch ping-pong,
Anila, for attentive and spirited proofreading
and the dedication of a loving sister,
Brian, for our delicious brainstorming and patience
with the earth science text editing,
Emerald Vallee, for an impromptu
Mentha piperita botanical drawing,
Yavanna, for font choice.

CONTENTS

continued

Preface

In writing about aromatherapy, crystals, and vibrational healing, I send out a wish to inspire, teach, and contribute to the balance that can be created in people and the world by consciously merging with natural elements.

If the spiritual evolves with the material, we have harmony. If the material evolves without the spiritual, we have disharmony and destruction. Harmony is about growth and development. Disharmony is about breaking systems apart.

Spirituality is not necessarily religion. I see the recognition of spirit in nature. Nature is the divine we can touch physically, our matrix, our mother, the support system for all life on earth.

There has never been a time of lasting peace on earth. We have not yet reached the Great Harmonics here. There has always been peace in the hearts of men, women and children, kept as a healthy seedling.

We are fortunate now to reach a time with a compelling pull to look in and become conscious. The time is now, to approach the creation of the Great Balance.

As long as we remember that we live on earth as the cells of a great organism, one with the environment, making amends, starting over fresh every day, healing differences and remembering the love, we will be following this pull of the necessary guidance towards a harmonious future.

We don't need technology to evolve as spirit on earth, but as we enjoy the wonderful advantages and excitement of our new technology, let us never forget our conscious relationship with the natural world.

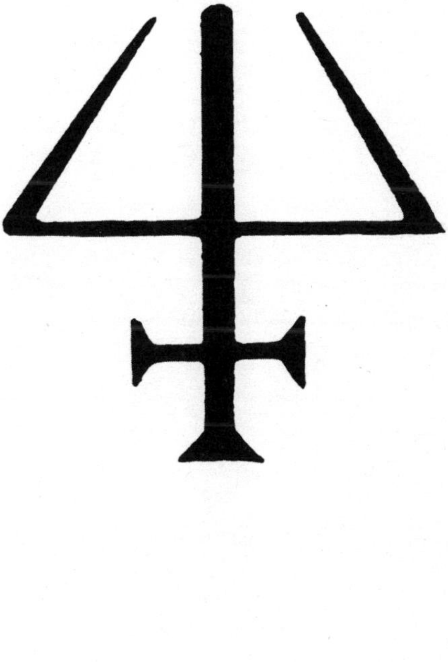

Alchemical Symbol for Essential Oil

PART ONE

Aromatherapy

...Greetings from our fragrant allies of the plant kingdom!
Inhaling their invisible treads as they transit between dimensions,
we feel the noble inspiration of a scented message... I am speaking of
the aroma from flowers, herbs, rind and resins that embody
the essence of a green Goddess... our fragrant earth.
~Kendra Grace

THE ESSENTIAL Q&A OF AROMATHERAPY

1. What is aromatherapy?

Aromatherapy is the art and science of using the therapeutic properties of essential oils to promote health and well-being of body, mind and emotions.

2. How long has aromatherapy been used?

Aromatherapy has been used since antiquity; and records exist of its use for at least 5,000 years. The Egyptians appear to have been the civilization most dedicated to the art and science of aromatherapy, using incense, perfume and cosmetics both spiritually and medicinally. We have proof of this in stone inscriptions, which gives us knowledge of their formulas and spiritual practices that used aromatic materials. Text is also found in the Vedic literature of India, 4,000 BCE, about the use of aromatic materials for medicine and cosmetics. This is what gave birth to a branch of the Ayurvedic system of medicine. China also has manuscripts as old as the Vedic ones, such as the Chinese medicine records of the Yellow Emperor, which describe uses for aromatic material. Mesopotamian civilizations used aromatic anointing as part of their spiritual practices. Later, Greeks and Romans, as well as the Arabian civilizations, inherited knowledge from the Egyptians and spread the use of aromatics throughout the Mediterranean region. In late 900 CE, an Arabian doctor and philosopher named Abu Ali Ibn Sina, known in the West as "Avicenna," developed the method of distillation of essential oils as we do it today, isolating the plant's aromatic material to obtain an extract. Later the knowledge was preserved in Europe, mostly by the French, and used by priests, alchemists, and women and men versed in the healing arts. It is also important to remember that primitive man used fumigations, the burning of aromatic plants, which can be seen as the first use of aromatherapy. Some form of aromatherapy has always been used and it is very unlikely that it will become extinct. In fact, with the refined technology we have available now, we are learning more and more about the therapeutic use of essential oils, and the role they play in enhancing of the quality of our lives.

3. How did aromatherapy fall into obscurity after being so popular in the ancient world?

With the Industrial Revolution, scientists investigated oils and the creation of synthetic compounds. Synthetic compounds became more prestigious, and "purity" very desirable. It reminds me of the prestige attached to white bread during a time when we lacked the understanding that fiber in bread is an important element. Now we are examining with more care the importance of trace elements.

During Renaissance times, the use of botanical oils in Europe was still practiced by alchemists and perfumers, which went hand in hand with herbalism and medicine.

It is my belief that the development of artificial oils has produced a massive olfactory confusion, disrupting the evolution of our former knowledge, with all of its implications. Archeologist and aromatic consultant John Steele, after completing specific research, concluded that our modern civilization is undergoing what he calls "sensory amnesia," a diminished awareness of smell. I think that synthetic molecules create a barrier in our perception of the signals we receive from nature, which we need in order to develop and realize our potential for holistic olfactory experience.

4. Why is aromatherapy so popular lately?

I believe humanity is ready for gentler and more holistic ways of healing and treating the earth and the body with more ecological awareness.

At the beginning of this new millennium, modern civilization is weary, and becoming increasingly mental and visual. The aromatic experience brings us down to earth and the body, creating more balance and helping to heal stress.

The pleasure that aromatherapy offers seems to be an easy route to open the mind, so that significant healing can take place.

People all over the world are leaning toward natural, alternative forms of medicine and cosmetic use.

5. What are essential oils?

Essential oils are very volatile substances produced from a botanical source. They are the concentrate of the aromatic molecules of a plant, or part of it; they can be considered the hormones of the plant, as they seem to control certain functions of plant life, including temperature and immune system. Essential oils are also similar to a hormone, as they can stimulate or slow down the biological functions of cell metabolism. Many people think of essential oils as the "spirit" of the plant.

6. What does the word "botanical" mean?

Often a misused word; when applied correctly, it means "of plant origin." A true botanical oil has not been created by synthesis in a laboratory, but distilled or extracted from the plant or its parts.

7. What are essential oils made of?

Essential oils are compositions of the basic organic elements carbon, oxygen and hydrogen, forming alcohols, aldehydes, esters, ketones, oxides, phenols and terpenes. An essential oil can contain from 10 to 200 components and other minor trace compounds, which are very difficult to analyze. Each essential oil has a more or less complex composition. Some are very simple, as in the case of sandalwood, containing 95 percent one compound, an alcohol named santalol, and 5 percent other components.

Some essential oils form very interesting and specific molecules that react against microorganisms such as bacteria and viruses. Such molecules sometimes can form a vitamin composition or a hormone-type chemical.

8. Are synthetic oils chemically the same as botanical oils?

There are chemists who like to proclaim that to be true; however, the botanical oils have proven by experience over thousands of years to have therapeutic or healing properties. One cannot say the same about synthetic oils. In fact, the opposite is true. (Refer to Jean Valnet, M.D., *The Practice of Aromatherapy*, p. 27.)

It is my belief that the oil from a plant that grew out of soil under sunshine and rain has an extremely different action to communicate to the human body than an oil that was born out of laboratory synthesis; that action is unique to a botanical oil because its balance is formed in a holistic situation.

Since our bodies are natural, living organisms, it makes sense that the extract from another natural, living organism would have a more harmonious and efficient interaction than a synthetic compound existing in no living matrix. Can we create ocean water in the lab to be the same as the ocean?

Synthetic oils may be too "pure," too simple a composition, not subtle enough to perform the complex functions that botanical oils exhibit. One may say that trace elements aren't important and that they make a composition "impure"; however, it is known that if humans occupying a space shuttle mission had to be away long from the Earth, surviving solely on synthetic compounds, then trace elements would become indispensable to sustain their lives.

Why do aromatherapists speak of essential oils having "life force"? I think that perhaps the minute and difficult-to-analyze trace elements may hold that section of the composition that pertains to what we call life force. Our systems can recognize and respond to the living balance (the natural signals) of the botanical oils. One of the important revelations of the recent aromatherapy rediscovery is the concept of essential oils as life-giving substances, which has been lost to the West since the industrial revolution.

9. Are "synthetic" and "adulterated" the same thing?

No. Synthetic and adulterated are not the same thing. Some botanical oils that are available commercially—for example, eucalyptus, lavender, and peppermint—have been put through a number of re-distillations. This process insures the so-called "purity" loved by the pharmaceutical and fragrance industry. For therapeutic uses, this purity actually ruins the original chemical balance of the oil, creating a greater percentage of its principal constituent than the original composition had. One can call these oils adulterated. The balance between active principle and trace elements is completely modified. Also, adulterated can mean an oil that is being sold as a pure essential oil but has been extended with vegetable oil or diethyl phthalate. Adulteration sometimes happens even before an oil enters the commercial market: at the distillation process, other plant material can enter the still as "fill" for a certain production that will be labeled as the principal plant being distilled.

There is also what is called "reconstruction" of oils. This is when some components of an essential oil are used to create a composition imitating another oil. This is the case of cheaper oil being used for the isolation of a component that can be used in the composition of more expensive oil. One example is the component geraniol, an alcohol found both in the cheaper oil of geranium and in the expensive rose oil. Although a reconstruction can utilize components from a botanical source, its finished result is a man-made composition in imitation of an original oil.

In the case of synthetic oils, compositions can be made in the lab without using plant sources.

10. How can one determine if an oil has been adulterated?

Become familiar with essential oils from a reputable source, oils that are distributed for the aromatherapy market. (See Appendix.)

If you have spent a good amount of time smelling essential oils, soon you will be able to distinguish the gentle feel of essential oils, in spite of their powerful smell. Oils that are redistilled, reconstructed or synthetic will be perceived as somewhat harsher. The more trained your nose becomes at smelling, the easier it will become to tell if the natural balance of a composition has been upset. One simple thing to remember: essential oils do not leave an oily residue on the surface of your skin. If the oil you are testing does, this oil has been extended with vegetable oil. Diethyl phthalate is a clear and odorless chemical commonly used to extend essential oils, and it will not leave an oily residue.

11. Are essential oils like vegetable oils?

Only that they are both from plant origin. Essential oils do not consist of fatty molecules, and vegetable oils do. Essential oils are aromatic and volatile, and vegetable oils are not. Essential oils evaporate rapidly, leaving no residue. Essential oils can vary in density—some have the consistency of water, and some can even be solid. They vary in color (clear, yellow, green, blue, orange, red, etc.) and have a powerful smell. They can be diluted in vegetable oil, alcohol or vinegar.

12. Can essential oils go rancid? Is there anything that can damage essential oils?

Rancidity, which presents itself as a foul smell or taste in vegetable oils, does not happen with essential oils. Essential oils can age as gracefully as good wines do, provided that they have been carefully preserved in a cool, dark place in tightly closed bottles when not in use.

Avoid exposing essential oils to direct light, heat, or contamination by another oil or substance. If these precautions have not been observed, there is the possibility that oils can become vulnerable to changes, and lose their potency, their life force.

13. How are essential oils produced?

By steam distillation (in most cases), by cold expression and by solvent extraction. The term *essential oils* is the definition of volatile oils resulting from steam distillation. The citrus-peel oils resulting from cold expression are known in the food industry as *essences*. Solvent extraction, generally the extract of flowers for the fragrance industry, yields the *absolute*.

14. Can you describe these methods further?

Cold expression can only be used in cases when the aromatic material can be easily obtained, and without the use of heat; all citrus oils go through this process that extracts the oil from the rind of the fruit by mechanical pressing.

In the case of flowers, so delicate that the aromatic material can be damaged by heat, the method of solvent extraction is used. *Rosa damascena*, orange blossom (neroli) and ylang ylang are the only flowers that can withstand the heat of steam distillation without damage, although the smell is not as close to the flower smell as with solvent extraction. All other plant materials can be processed by hot water/steam distillation, in a still (an apparatus consisting of a vat, a tank for holding the plants, and another for producing steam from water). After essential oils flow from plants into the hot water, the temperature is lowered to separate the oil, which rises to the surface and is decanted away.

15. Can you explain solvent extraction further?

Solvent extraction is a method that uses hydrocarbon-type solvents, products from the petrochemical industry such as acetone, hexane, butane, or propane. It can produce a truer-to-nature smell of the flowers than hot water steam distillation can. What is obtained is a creamy solid called the *concrete*. This concrete contains a percentage of flower wax, which in turn is further refined, and the petrochemical solvent is removed by ethanol alcohol to produce the final substance of the process, the *absolute*. Absolutes can be extracted from other plant parts, but are mostly extracted from flowers, and this absolute is called *precious flower oil*. Steam-distilled rose and orange blossoms are also called precious flower oils.

16. How are concretes and absolutes used in aromatherapy?

Concretes and absolutes are produced for the fragrance industry. These oils have traces of solvent residues, thus are not desirable for use in medical aromatherapy, as oils can be prescribed to be taken internally.

I have used these flower oils extensively in psycho-aromatherapy for their aroma, and I feel that a massage oil or a skin care blend with a small amount of these precious flower oils does no harm. The precious flower oils have therapeutic properties as well, as the long, extensive history of their use demonstrates.

17. How did people in the past obtain oils from the flowers?

Oils were obtained by an old method, now abandoned, called *enfleurage*. Enfleurage was a process using animal fat. It consisted of placing flower petals on top of a layer of fat, to saturate the fat with the aromatic material. The flowers had to be removed at the end of the day and a fresh new layer applied, until saturation had reached desired strength. The aromatic oil would be used with the fatty base. In ancient times, aromatic oils were made by infusion, the placement of herbs and flowers into vegetable oils. These mixtures were exposed to the sun for a period of time.

18. Is there any modern method that produces a true-to-nature smell of flowers in oil that is also free of residue?

Extraction by liquid carbon dioxide is one modern method that produces a true smell that is also free of residue. It is performed just above room temperature. Since carbon dioxide can act as an inert gas, it does not react with aromatic material during extraction and leaves no residue. Extraction by carbon dioxide uses very sophisticated and expensive equipment, developed to supply food-grade oils to the food industry.

In 1987, Dr. Peter Wilde developed an extraction process called *phytonics*. This is performed at cold temperatures, using possibly the cleanest technology available today. Environmentally friendly, non-ozone-depleting hydroflourocarbons are used to deliver a product of pharmaceutical quality. This extraction method is demonstrated in my documentary *Precious Essence*, available through my website (see Appendix).

19. *What is the difference between flower essences and flower oils?*

Flower essences are vibrational remedies, created by placing flowers in water and exposing them to sun or moonlight to extract an etheric imprint of the flower. The English doctor Edward Bach developed flower essences in 1930. These remedies are aimed at the etheric and electromagnetic field of the human body in order to heal illnesses of a subtle order, emotional and mental. Precious flower oils are a physical extract of the aromatic material of the flower, and they can affect the mind and emotions at the same time as their therapeutic properties address conditions in the physical body.

20. *Can aromatherapy interfere with homeopathic treatment?*

There is no "scientifically satisfying" answer to whether aromatherapy interferes with homeopathic treatment. Homeopathy is a vibrational medicine method using a holistic system of treatment. Because it is still not easily understood by the general public, people react extra-sensitively about it. Thought and emotion are not physical, but they can affect matter. It is a usual agreement that an emotion can make the physical body sick. Why then, can not only powerful essential oils but also a powerful emotion interfere with a homeopathic treatment? Even more significant would then be the *thought* that essential oils would affect the homeopathic treatment. French author Marguerite Maury believed in the synergy of homeopathic and aromatherapy treatments. (See Marguerite Maury's *Guide to Aromatherapy*, ch. 10.)

My thought on this is that if both treatments are intentionally used at once, the doctor prescribing homeopathy should also know aromathcrapy.

Say someone is under homeopathic treatment and is having an aromatherapy massage. What happens is going to depend in large on the influence of this person's beliefs and emotions about using both. If the homeopathy treatment is for an illness that is causing the individual a lot of emotional stress, I can only conclude by logic that if essential oils are being used to sedate the nervous system, it is not going against the intention and action of the homeopathic treatment, but only enhancing its action.

21. Are there different types of aromatherapy practices?

Aromatherapy is naturally divided into three distinct fields: medicinal use, cosmetic use, and psychology or psychotherapy.

The **medical branch** of aromatherapy involves in-depth study of how the properties of each oil affect organs and internal tissue to promote healing. Oils can be taken internally under the direction of an expert, as certain oils can be toxic to the organism and must be used with experienced precision. Oils in dilution are applied on the body through the skin by massage, to address internal or external dysfunctions, or treat conditions such as bacterial or viral infections. Oils can address conditions in the internal organs using gelatin capsules or suppositories.

In the foreground of this work are France and England, where a number of medical doctors are using aromatherapy in hospitals. In France, aromatherapy is offered as a course in medical school.

The **cosmetic branch** of aromatherapy practice is in the hands of estheticians and massage therapists who use essential oils in skin care, hair and other beauty treatments, relaxation and spa therapies. An increasing number of cosmetic companies are now using plant-source essential oils in their cosmetic formulations.

In **psycho-aromatherapy**, the use of essential oils is applied to psychotherapy. This involves the study of the relationship between memory/emotion and scent, and how that can be used to improve an individual's emotional/mental condition. One can call it "therapy by aroma."

22. Can you say a word about the toxicity of essential oils?

The first thing to remember is that although essential oils are natural, botanical substances, this does not guarantee safety. Fortunately, the most poisonous plants are not aromatic and the majority of essential oils (85-90 percent) are quite safe to use.

The next thing to remember is the quantity and the concentration; for example, how much essential oil is diluted in a vegetable oil to be used either internally or externally.

Essential oils are 70 times more concentrated than their aromatic components in the plant that they were extracted from. Essential oils should only be ingested in precise dosages. Care should also be taken in the dilution of oils for external use, and the frequency of application.

Robert Tisserand has studied this subject extensively and in his *The Essential Oil Safety Data Manual* he classified essential oils hazards into three categories:

Toxicity—different degrees of poisoning.

Irritation—inflammation of mucus membranes or skin. (Frequency of application in relation to the body's response to irritation is important here.)

Sensitization—allergic reaction, mostly manifesting on the skin, involving the immune system. Sensitization can occur with small amounts and few (or a single) applications.

Again, remember that the majority of oils are perfectly harmless and poisoning has only been reported in cases of excessive overdose, such as 50 to 200 times over a safe dose of a toxic oil. Ingestion of essential oils in the form of spices with toxic aromatic material has marked quite a long path in history. Common sense concludes that the therapeutic use of essential oils will not give rise to the unexpected side effects we risk in the case of comparably new, shortly-tested synthetic chemicals.

23. Why are toxic oils produced and what are the most toxic oils?

Some toxic oils are very powerful therapeutically. For example, oil that can be an irritant to a certain organ, can also be used to treat this organ, in the right concentrations. It has been documented that low concentrations are very effective.

Below are some of the most common toxic oils in descending order of hazardous effects:

Toxicity:

Mustard, Rue, Savin, Horseradish, Pennyroyal, Mugwort, Hyssop, Wormwood, Wintergreen, Thyme, Fennel.

Skin sensitivity:

Bergamot, Clove, Cinnamon, Cumin, Pine, Oregano, Sassafras, Savory, Juniper. (Leaves and twigs only. Juniper berry oil is not toxic.)

24. Why is aromatherapy important in skin care?

The life-giving support and cell regeneration capabilities of essential oils give them remarkable utility in skin care.

Most essential oils have an antiseptic effect, acting against bacteria. Their amazing ability to penetrate creates an obvious advantage in skin care, not only to balance different skin conditions and treat acne, but also to serve as natural preservatives in cosmetics. Since some essential oils have compounds that can be compared to hormones, they have the ability to stimulate or calm our own hormones, serving to regulate the functions of the skin.

25. Can acne be cured with essential oils?

Acne is complex, not just skin deep. Stress, genetics, and diet are major factors in creating the imbalances that promote acne. The aromatic experience of essential oils reduces stress via relaxing the mind and body.

Certain oils have properties that can improve skin circulation, which is usually poor in skins with acne. An oil that is a strong bactericidal, such as lemon, can help a skin with acne diminish the production of bacteria and neutralize the waste products caused by it. (See Exotic Kitchen Recipes, page 118.)

26. Why are scent and the sense of smell associated with memory and emotion?

Fairly extensive research has been done in Europe, Japan, United States and Russia on the association of memory, emotion and the sense of smell. Internal nasal membranes contain olfactory receptors, but the olfactory bulb is inside the cranial area. Our sense of smell is processed in the brain, below the hypothalamus, in the cortex, where memory and emotion are processed. This part of our brain, nicknamed "the smell brain," the rhinencephalon, was one of the first areas to develop.

In primitive man, as well as in modern man, information needed from memory and emotion strongly depends on the sense of smell to trigger action and behavior regarding the gathering of food, hunting, migration, escape, sexual interaction, and the processing of more subtle information.

27. How do memory, emotion, and scent association relate to aromatherapy?

Presently, there are a small number of psycho-aromatherapists, myself included, who are using the memory/emotion and scent associations of essential oils as a tool to apply different methods of therapy, to heal patients' emotional and mental conditions. This practice is of great use in clinical psychotherapy, for hospice and hospital patients, and for substance-addiction patients in rehabilitation centers.

28. How and when was the word aromatherapy first used?

The term *aromatherapy* was first coined in France by a chemist named René-Maurice Gattefossé who, by accident, rediscovered the therapeutic properties of essential oils. In 1928, Gattefossé was working in his family's perfumery lab when he got a severe burn on his hand. He dipped his hands in a pan of organic lavender oil that was sitting close by. He noticed that the lavender oil stopped the spread of burn damage that was developing on his tissues. The burn healed rapidly and with little scarring. He was fascinated, and began researching the antiseptic and antibiotic properties of essential oils. Later his studies attracted interest in France, Germany and Switzerland, gathering a small group in the scientific community in Europe, among who are Dr. Jean Valnet, Dr. Jean Claude Lapraz, Dr. Daniel Pénoël, and research scientist Pierre Franchomme, who continue to work with medical aromatherapy.

Forty years later Robert Tisserand succeeded in spreading the word *aromatherapy* in Europe and the United States by publishing his popular book, *The Art of Aromatherapy*.

29. What is the future of aromatherapy?

As most societal accomplishments often begin with one individual, it is easy to observe that the natural path aromatherapy is taking started with the rediscovery and growth in knowledge from Gattefossé, reached a group of scientific researchers, and now is appearing in the societies of the world in many different forms.

Environmental fragrancing seems to be one of the important avenues of action affecting society, which is going to teach us about the power of the aromatic experience in many areas of our lives, all over the world. Avid research and current applications active now in Japan use the therapeutic properties of plant-source essential oils in the workplace, using modern techniques of diffusing aromatic molecules in office buildings and homes. In England the essential oil of lavender is a deodorizer in the subway transportation system. In France, doctors have found that the dispersion of essential oils in hospitals helps to control the proliferation of airborne germs and viruses.

The Essential Oils

The list of essential oils in this chapter contains the most important oils for the beginner to learn and use, and the ones most immediately available through most stores selling essential oils.

My sources of information for writing this chapter were the works of Dr. Kurt Schnaubelt, Dr. Pénoël, Pierre Franchomme, Robert Tisserand, Julia Lawless, Dr. Jean Valnet, and others. For further study and reputable essential oil labels for aromatherapy, refer to the Appendix.

All essential oils lend themselves to a wide variety of actions that describe their properties. This chapter lists only the most prominent actions for each oil described, as a quick reference. See the description of these properties at the end of this chapter for further information.

Below is a list of the oils included in this chapter:

Basil	Mint, peppermint
Bergamot	Orange blossom (Neroli)
Chamomile	Rose
Eucalyptus	Rosemary
Frankincense	Sage, clary
Geranium	Sandalwood
Jasmine	Tea tree
Lavender	Ylang ylang
Lemon	

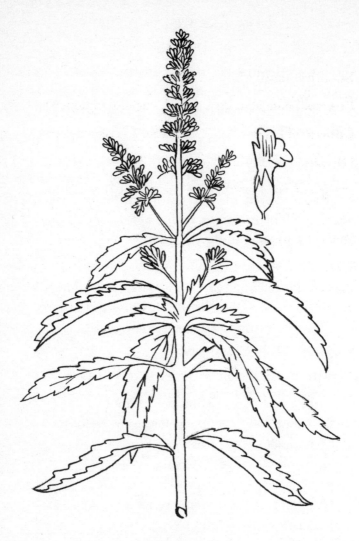

BASIL
Ocimum basilicum

BASIL
Ocimum basilicum

Botanical family: Labiatae.

Principal components: Linalol, eugenol, limonene.

Climate of origin: Tropical. Native to Asia and Africa.

Oil extracted from: Leaves and flowers of herb.

Produced in: Egypt, France, India, Pacific Islands, United States, Brazil.

Blending class: Top note.

Characteristics: Yellow oil, fresh, herbaceous "green" odor, bittersweet taste. Blends well with clary sage, geranium, lavender, lime. Used in perfumery and the food industry.

History & lore: Used widely in India's Ayurvedic medicine known as *tulsi*, to treat bronchitis, coughs, flu and stomach ailments. Also used as an antidote against snake and insect bites, taken internally or applied on the skin.

Basil has been associated with the scorpion, the planet Mars and the element Fire.

Therapeutic properties: Relieves smooth muscle spasms, so is indicated for nausea; stimulant for the mind in depressive states; insect repellent and mosquito bite relief. Think of basil when you feel nervousness that affects your stomach giving you pangs and nausea; also think of basil when your mind feels gray and slow and your mental focus is failing you. Avoid in the first trimester of pregnancy.

Actions: Antispasmodic, cephalic, stimulant, antidepressant.

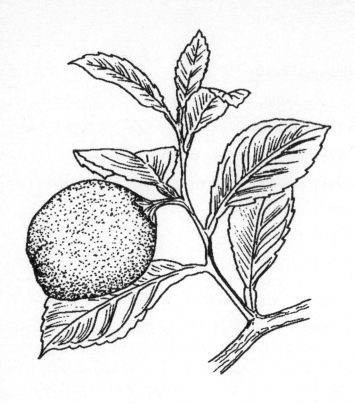

BERGAMOT

Citrus bergamia

BERGAMOT
Citrus bergamia

Botanical family: Rutaceae.

Principal Components: Linalyl acetate, linalol, sesquiterpene bergapten.

Climate of origin: Tropical; native to Asia.

Oil extracted from: Rind of fruit of small tree.

Produced in: Italy and the Ivory Coast.

Blending class: Top note.

Characteristics: Light green oil with a fresh, sweet scent. Blends well with all citrus and flower oils, and with lavender, geranium and juniper.

History & lore: Bergamot oil has been widely used in Italian folk medicine. It was first sold in Italy in the town of Bergamo, from which its name is derived.

One of its components, a furocoumarins named bergapten, has been found to cause skin pigmentation—staining skin if exposed to sunlight—with possible sensitization even in dilution.

It is one of the ingredients of the classic eau-de cologne and is widely used in the food and fragrance industry.

Ruled by the Sun and the element Fire.

Therapeutic properties: Bergamot oil has been used for treating infection of the mucus membranes of the mouth, throat, respiratory, urinary tracts and female organs (used in douches and sitz baths). It is useful as an antiseptic against infection caused by organisms such as gonococcus, staphylococcus, coli, meningococcus and diphtheria bacillus.

Actions: Analgesic, antiseptic, cicatrisant, deodorant, sedative.

CHAMOMILE

ROMAN CHAMOMILE
Chamaemelum nobile

Botanical family: Compositae.

Principal components: Pinocarvone, farnesol, pinene, nerolidol, cineol.

Climate of origin: Temperate to cold climates. Native to southwest Europe.

Oil extracted from: Entire herb when flowering.

Produced in: Belgium, England, France, Hungary, Italy.

Blending class: Top note.

Characteristics: Pale blue liquid when new, turning yellow with age. Apple-like scent, sweet and warm, bitter taste. Blends well with clary sage, geranium, jasmine, lavender and neroli.

History & lore: Used throughout the Mediterranean region, it was called the "plant's physician," from the popular belief that this herb kept other garden plants healthy. In the Middle Ages it was planted on the garden path, so that when stepped on it would release its apple-like scent. Associated with the Moon and the element Water, it was one of the Saxon's nine sacred herbs.

Therapeutic properties: Helpful as a sedative in nervous states having to do with physical impact such as shock, blows, or injuries affecting the nervous system. Wonderful for calming infants. A good remedy for asthma with nervous origin, and for intestinal parasites.

Actions: Analgesic, antispasmodic, cicatrisant, hepatic, sedative.

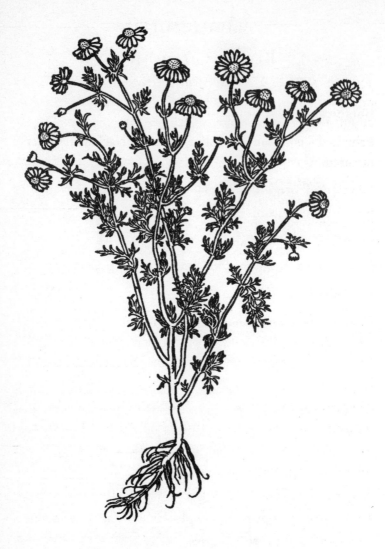

GERMAN CHAMOMILE
Matricaria recutita

CHAMOMILE, GERMAN
Matricaria recutita, blue chamomile

This chamomile contains chamazulene, or azulene, as its principal component. A very powerful substance consisting of anti-inflammatory blue crystals, azulene is formed as the essential oil is distilled from the flowers. Think of chamomile to counteract the inflamed, red tissue (internally or externally) that produces swelling, bruises, rashes, rheumatic pains, sore muscles and teething aches. German chamomile is also called "blue" chamomile.

In appearance it is ink blue. An absolute (a fixative with a more viscous consistency) is also produced from the flowers. *Matricaria recutita* has a stronger odor and is warmer and sweeter than Roman chamomile.

Climate of Origin: Temperate. Native to Europe and northwest Asia. The oil is currently produced in Hungary and Germany.

Therapeutic Properties: Tonic for the digestive system, used to treat dyspepsia and gastrointestinal ulcers. Also used to treat inflamed conditions on the skin such as acne and dermatosis, and internal organ tissue inflammations.

Actions: Anti-inflammatory, antispasmodic, anti-allergic, tonic and cicatrisant.

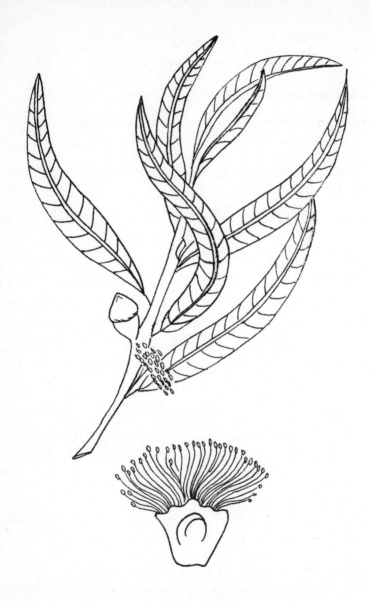

EUCALYPTUS
Eucalyptus globulus

Eucalyptus
Eucalyptus globulus

Botanical family: Myrtaceae.

Principal components: Eucalyptol, cineol, pinene, limonene, terpenene.

Climate of origin: Tropical, sub-tropical to dry temperate. Native of Australia.

Oil extracted from: Leaves of large tree.

Produced in: Spain, Portugal, Brazil, California.

Blending class: Top note; not recommended for perfumery.

Characteristics: White to yellow liquid with somewhat harsh, strong odor; mildly bitter taste; blends well with lavender, rosemary, lemon. Used extensively in the pharmaceutical industry for a wide variety of medical preparations, and as a flavoring agent in the food industry.

History & lore: Used in Australia for respiratory problems and, secondarily, on the skin. The leaves are smoked for asthma and applied on burns and open wounds for fast healing. Ruled by the planet Saturn and the element Earth.

Therapeutic properties: The eucalyptus oil can be used in massage blends to relieve muscular aches and joint pain, and to improve poor circulation.

Eucalyptus is a remedy for outbreaks of herpes simplex (lip sores). It can be applied neat to shorten the virus outbreak, and to relieve pain. In cases of bronchitis, it is used in inhalations or applied diluted in massage on the lung area (back of chest).

Actions: Analgesic, anti-viral, expectorant, stimulant.

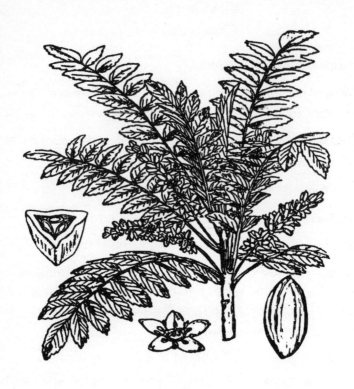

Frankincense
Boswellia carterii

FRANKINCENSE
Boswellia carterii

Botanical family: Burseraceae.

Principal components: Terpenene, pinene, dipentene, limonene, thujene, cymene, incensole, octylacetate.

Climate of origin: Subtropical, dry climates. Native of the Red Sea region.

Oil extracted from: Gum resin from small tree.

Produced in: South Arabia, Somalia, Ethiopia, China.

Blending class: Base note.

Characteristics: Clear to yellow liquid with a woody/spicy odor. Used in the pharmaceutical and perfume industries, in the manufacture of incense, and to a smaller degree in the food industry as a flavoring agent.

History & lore: Frankincense was highly regarded in the ancient civilizations of the Middle East and Africa. One of the gifts of the wise men to the infant Christ, it was considered as valuable as gold. Frankincense was of primary importance in commerce. The Egyptians used frankincense for their famous rejuvenating facial masks.

In the Middle Ages frankincense was used in hospitals to fumigate or "smoke" patients suffering from evil spirits (madness).

In India, it was used for treatment of all kinds of internal and external infections. Frankincense is ruled by the Sun and the element Fire.

Therapeutic properties: Treatment of infected wounds. It is a strong astringent, useful in inhalations for catarrhal conditions of the lungs. Also used to draw out genito-urinary tract infections.

In skin care, frankincense is used for mature skin and wrinkle formulas.

Soothing effect on the mind and emotions.

Actions: Antiseptic, astringent, cicatrisant, sedative.

GERANIUM
Pelargonium graveolens

Botanical family: Geraniaceae.

Principal components: Geraniol, citronellol, linalol, limonene.

Climate of origin: Subtropical. Native of South Africa.

Oil extracted from: The whole plant when flowering.

Produced In: China, Madagascar.

Blending class: Middle note.

Characteristics: Green liquid with strong sweet/fresh odor and bitter taste. Blends well with almost any oil, especially with lavender, rose, sandalwood, basil and all citrus oils. Used in the fragrance and food industry.

History & lore: Since antiquity, geranium has been well regarded for treating all female complaints, such as excessive menstruation, hot flashes, and vaginitis. Ruled by the planet Venus and the element Earth.

Therapeutic properties: Geranium is a stimulant of the adrenal cortex, which produces sex hormones. It can act as a balancing stimulant for female organs and the nervous system and relieve the pain of vaginal herpes sores and other inflamed conditions of the vaginal mucus membranes. It is used for eczema treatments and as an insect repellent. Analgesic and astringent, it is also helpful in breast engorgement and hemorrhoids.

Actions: Analgesic, astringent, cicatrisant, haemostatic.

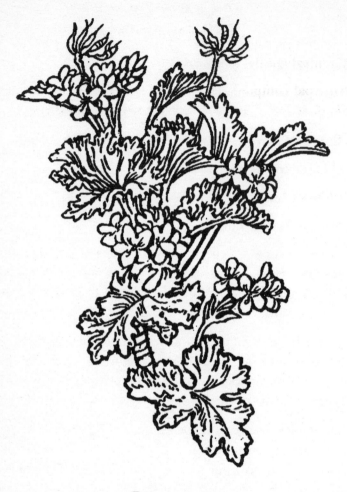

GERANIUM
Pelargonium graveolens

Jasmine
Jasminum officinale

Botanical family: Jasminaceae.

Principal components: Benzyl acetate, benzyl alcohol, cis-jasmone, linalol, farnesol, indole, methyl jasmonate.

Climate of origin: Native to China and Asia.

Oil extracted from: Flowers of shrub.

Produced in: India, France, Morocco, Egypt, Japan, China, Italy.

Blending class: Base note.

Characteristics: Reddish-brown, viscous liquid with a inebriating sweet floral scent; blends well with most essences.

History & lore: Jasmine has long been a favorite of Eastern nations and has an established reputation as an aphrodisiac and indispensable ingredient in sensual massage to relax the body. In China, jasmine flowers are used to scent tea. The flowers must be picked at night during their yearly season, and in India jasmine is nicknamed "moonlight of the grove." Jasmine is one of the most expensive botanical oils, an absolute used in high-class perfumery.

Ruled by the planet Jupiter and the element Fire.

Therapeutic properties: Jasmine has a relaxing effect on the nervous system and has been reported to increase alpha brain waves.

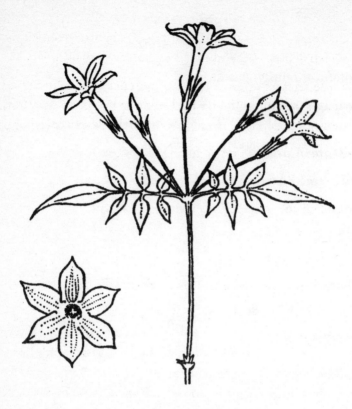

JASMINE
Jasminum officinale

In the West, jasmine has been used as a tonic for the male and female reproductive organs, to ease labor pains, to remedy after-birth depression, and to help with the flow of milk.

Jasmine seems to have a marked presence in modifying depressive states of mind and in stimulating positive emotions. Excellent for depression and grief after death of a loved one.

Actions: Antidepressant, antispasmodic, aphrodisiac, galactogogue, sedative.

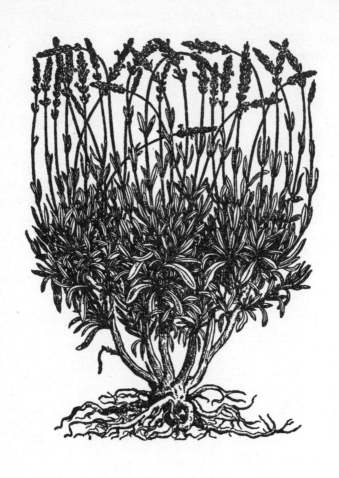

LAVENDER
Lavandula officinalis

LAVENDER
Lavandula officinalis

There are many varieties of the genus *lavandula*, cultivated all over the world. *Lavandula officinalis* is the general term to describe the genus. The most known varieties, *Lavandula angustifolia* or *Lavandula vera*, and *Lavandula latifolia*, by bee pollination create the hybrid lavender known as *lavandin*.

All of these lavenders are different "chemotypes" meaning their natural chemistry varies slightly in composition, and therefore they also vary in therapeutic properties. However, all have a sedating effect on the central nervous system and can be used for antiseptic and deodorant actions.

Botanical family: Labiatae.

Principal components: Linalol, lavandulyl acetate, linalyl acetate, lavandulol, cineol, limonene, terpineol.

Climate of origin: Temperate, dry. Native to the Mediterranean region.

Oil extracted from: Entire herb when flowering.

Produced in: A variety of climates, temperate to cold. France, Spain, Italy, England, Bulgaria, Australia, Greece, Russia. The best oil comes from the French Alps.

Blending class: Top note.

Characteristics: By steam distillation, a clear liquid with a powerful herbal/floral odor, with a mildly bitter taste. By solvent extraction, an absolute, a thicker, deep green oil with a sweeter odor; blends well with most floral, citrus and herbal oils. Widely used in the perfume industry.

History & lore: Lavender was first established in the western world by the Romans, who used lavender extensively in their bathing rituals. The word is derived from the Latin word *lavare*, meaning "to wash."

Lavender has a long-standing tradition in the preparation of sachets, to scent linens and in floral waters. In birthing and convalescent rooms, lavender flowers were burned to create a aura of cleanness and to please deities.

Lavender is ruled by the planet Mercury and the element Air.

Therapeutic properties: Lavender is known as "the universal oil" because it lends itself to so many different uses. It is wonderful as an anti-stress agent in a bath to relax body, mind and emotion. It is a remedy for migraines, insomnia and nervous depression. Lavender is a strong, non-toxic antiseptic that can be applied neat on cuts and burns to prevent infection and help promote fast formation of scar tissue to close a wound, and can be used to treat anal fistula. A mild sedative, lavender soothes skin suffering from overexposure to the sun; also a mosquito and spider bite relief and repellent. In childbirth, lavender is very helpful to relax the mother during contractions. It is a mild sedative in infant's massage oil to relax its neuro/muscular system after birth.

Actions: Analgesic, antiseptic, antitoxic, cicatrisant, deodorant, sedative.

LEMON
Citrus limon

Botanical family: Rutaceae.

Principal components: Limonene, linalol, pinene, geraniol, citral, terpenene, citronellal.

Climate of origin: Temperate. Native to Asia.

Oil extracted from: Rind of fruit of small tree.

Produced in: Spain, Portugal, Italy, Brazil, California.

Blending class: Top note.

Characteristics: A greenish-yellow liquid with a mild and refreshing citrus note, and a sharp, tart taste. Blends well with geranium, lavender, eucalyptus, neroli, rose, sandalwood.

It is used extensively by the fragrance, pharmaceutical and food industries.

History & lore: In European Latin countries and South America, a household does not function without lemons. The juice of the lemon is used as a bactericide, to soak and wash meat prior to cooking, and as a drink to treat infectious diseases and to reduce fever.

Therapeutic properties: The essential oil of lemon is the most powerful antiseptic of all essences. It is a good inhalation remedy for respiratory tract infections during a cold or flu, or as a tea for food poisoning.

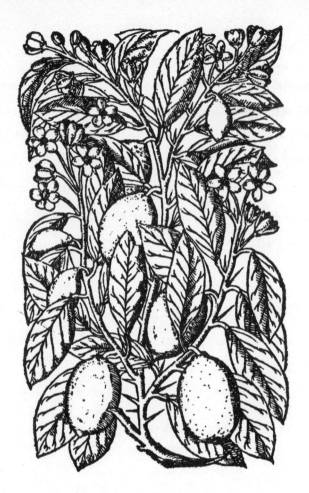

LEMON
Citrus limon

Lemon has a tonic and detoxifying effect on the gastric mucus membranes; it promotes a healthy flow of urine and stimulates the production of white blood cells. It is thinning to the blood, and therefore helpful to those suffering from high blood pressure.

Lemon also has a neutralizing action on the liver and helps those who are anemic because of liver malfunction.

Actions: Antiseptic, antitoxic, bactericidal, diuretic, febrifuge, haemostatic, hypotensive, anti-anemic.

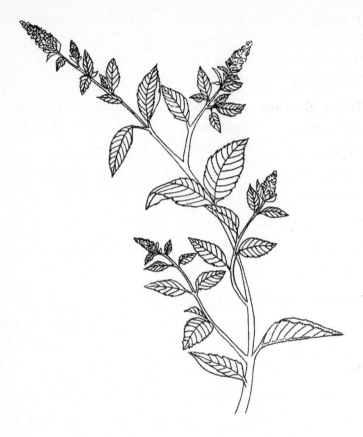

Mint, Peppermint
Mentha piperita

Mint, Peppermint
Mentha piperita

Botanical family: Labitae.

Principal components: Menthol, limonene, cineol, menthyl acetate.

Climate of origin: The peppermint that is cultivated now is a hybrid of other mints developed in England. Possibly, it is original to the Mediterranean region.

Oil extracted from: Entire plant when flowering.

Produced in: All over the world; most importantly in England, France, United States, China.

Blending class: Top note.

Characteristics: A light green or yellow liquid with a powerfully penetrating, zesty, camphor-like odor. It blends well with lemon, eucalyptus, lavender and rosemary.

Used by the pharmaceutical, food and fragrance industries.

History & lore: There is record of peppermint tracing as far back as being cultivated by the Egyptians. In Greek mythology, there is the mention of a sensual nymph called Mentha who became dear to the God Pluto, who transformed her into the herb peppermint after displays of jealousy by his wife, Goddess Persephone.

Ruled by the planet Mercury and the element Air.

Therapeutic properties: Principal aromatherapeutic remedy for flatulence, indigestion and colic.

Useful for the respiratory system in the form of inhalations to relieve asthma, bronchitis, head colds, and dry coughs. Peppermint can be diluted into a massage oil to be applied locally to lungs (back of chest). Good for fainting spells and mental fatigue.

Actions: Antispasmodic, analgesic, carminative, expectorant, vasoconstrictor, cephalic.

Orange Blossom (Neroli)
Citrus aurantium

Botanical family: Rutaceae.

Climate of origin: Temperate. Native to China, grows well in dry soil such as in the Mediterranean region.

Principal components: Linalol, linalyl acetate, limonene, nerolidol, nerol, indole, pinene, citral, jasmone, geraniol.

Oil extracted from: Flowers of the bitter orange tree.

Produced in: France, Tunisia, Italy, Morocco.

Blending class: Top note.

Characteristics: The absolute, by solvent extraction, is a reddish-brown, viscous liquid with a wonderfully sweet "high pitch" and mildly narcotic scent; essential oils have a bitter taste; blends well with all essences, especially floral and citrus oils. The steam-distilled oil is light yellow in color, and is mostly known as Neroli. Very expensive oil used in high-class perfumery.

History & lore: Used in China since antiquity for scenting cosmetics. Traditionally a favorite of many countries for bridal bouquets and headdresses. This custom is attributed to the fact that the pretty smell of orange flowers can sedate the bride on her wedding day. Often a tranquilizing tea from the leaves and flowers of the bitter orange tree would also be given to the bride prior to attending the ceremony.

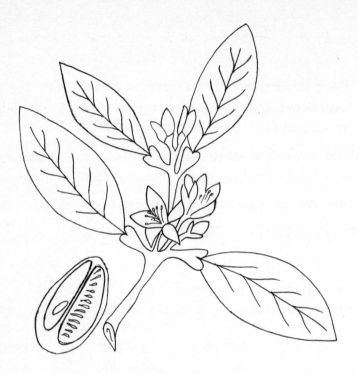

Orange Blossom (Neroli)
Citrus aurantium

The nickname "neroli" probably came from the princess of Nerola who was the first one to set the trend of perfuming leather gloves with the perfume of orange blossoms.

In Arabian countries, the orange blossom water, a by-product of the flower distillation process, is used as a digestive drinking water and also in the preparation of fine pastries.

Ruled by the Sun and the element Fire.

Therapeutic properties: If lemon oil is the most important aromatherapy antiseptic, neroli is the most important sedative. Neroli has an action on the heart, slowing cardiac contractions in palpitations and spasm. It is of great value in therapies dealing with sudden shock or unbearable stress, as in cases of hysteria, anxiety, fear of death, grief, and strong emotions affecting the heart. Neroli can be used in cases of nervous diarrhea, and it helps eliminate intestinal gas and colic. A relaxing bath can be made to treat nervous depression.

Neroli is non-toxic. The diluted orange blossom water is an excellent soothing drink for infants' colic and for insomnia.

Actions: Antidepressant, aphrodisiac, cordial, digestive, hypotensor, sedative.

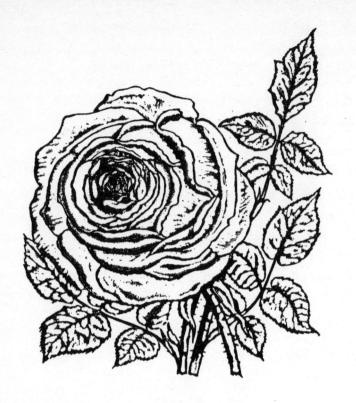

ROSE
Rosa maroc

Rose

Among more than 10,000 varieties of rose, three distinct varieties are cultivated for rose oil production: *Rosa centifolia, Rosa gallica,* and *Rosa damascena.*

The rose known as *Rose maroc,* or Cabbage rose, is a hybrid rose that combines the pink *Rosa centifolia* with the red *Rosa gallica,* and is used for the production of the true extract of rose, the absolute.

Rosa gallica was the apothecary's garden rose, widely used by monks and alchemists in the medicinal preparations of early Europe. *Rosa Damascena*, a fragile and fragrant variety, is cultivated in Bulgaria and Turkey for the production of steam-distilled *otto*, the essential oil of rose.

Note that in India a perfume named aytar, a combination of rose and sandalwood, became famous all over the world. Do not confuse this with the name *otto* that refers to the pure steam-distilled rose oil.

Rosa centifolia

Botanical family: Rosaceae.

Principal constituents: Phenyl ethanol, geranial, nerol, citronellol, stearopten, farnesol, plus hundreds of others in minute traces.

Climate of origin: Temperate.

Blending class: Base note.

Produced in: Morocco, France, England, Italy, China.

Characteristics: The otto is a light yellow liquid with a warm, sweet odor; the absolute is a reddish-orange, denser oil with a richer, sweet aroma. Blends well with most essential oils.

History & lore: Used extensively during Medieval times as a "cure-all" medicine; still of prime importance in Ayurvedic and Chinese medicine. The Greeks regarded the rose as the flower of Aphrodite (Venus), Goddess of beauty and love. The most feminine of all scents, the perfume of rose has been used as an aphrodisiac and for magic rituals throughout history. Since early times the rose essence has been known to have a therapeutic action on the heart and womb, and can regulate excessive bleeding.

Ruled by the planet Venus and the element Earth.

Therapeutic properties: Rose oil can be used for balancing female sexual organ disorders, hemorrhages, mastitis, stress-related problems, impotence, frigidity, irritable and sensitive skin, eczema, broken capillaries, poor circulation, headaches, hay fever and liver disorders.

Actions: Aphrodisiac, astringent, cordial, galactagogue, haemostatic, hepatic, rubefacient, sedative, uterine.

Rosa Damascena

Botanical family: Rosaceae.

Principal constituents: Citronellol, geraniol, nerol, stearopten, phenyl ethanol, farnesol and many others.

Climate of origin: Temperate; native to the Far East.

Oil extracted from: Flowers of shrub.

Produced in: Bulgaria, France, Turkey.

Blending class: Base note.

Characteristics: A light yellow, sometimes faintly green liquid that can solidify at room temperature. It has a tart/sweet narcotic-like scent, very powerful and not commonly pleasant to the unaccustomed person in its undiluted form. One drop or less of this otto can go a long way in a blend. Bulgarian rose otto is one of the most expensive essential oils. It takes from 30 to 60 roses to produce a single drop of rose oil. Used in high-class perfumery.

History & lore: This cultivated rose may have been developed in Persia in ancient times. Legend tells of a princess' wedding where the garden was cut with canals. For the ceremony, roses were placed on the water of these canals. With the heat, rose essence appeared floating visibly on the surface of the water. Supposedly, after this incident, the Persians were the first to develop a distillation process to obtain the rose oil. This rose is now cultivated in Morocco, France, Italy and China.

For properties and actions see *Rosa centifolia*.

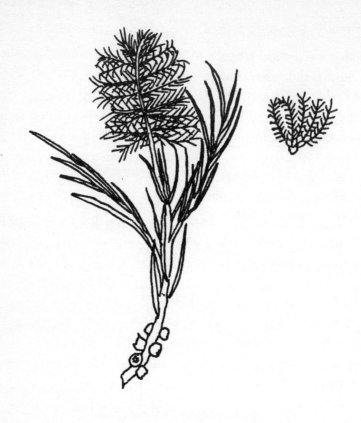

Rosemary
Rosmarinus officinalis

Rosemary
Rosmarinus officinalis

Botanical family: Labiatae.

Principal constituents: Pinene, limonene, linalol, cineol, borneol, camphene, terpineol.

Climate of origin: Temperate dry, desert. Native to the Mediterranean region.

Oil extracted from: Entire plant when flowering.

Produced in: France, Tunisia, Spain, California, China.

Blending class: Middle note.

Characteristics: Clear liquid with a penetrating green fresh/herbal scent; relatively mellow minty taste; blends well with basil, peppermint, lemon, and lavender.

History & lore: The influence of the piercing scent of rosemary has been recognized since early times in the European medicine as a remedy for "weakness of the brain." In France, fumigations (burning to cause an aromatic smoke; smudging) were prepared in hospitals to get rid of "evil spirits."

Rosemary tea was used to awaken the senses and liven the memory.

Rosemary facial wash was used as a beautifying agent, tinctures of it were used to darken the hair, and this herb was often present in culinary uses, for flavoring meats and other dishes.

The mere presence of this plant was believed to drive away fever. Used extensively in medieval magic rituals. In ancient Greece it was regarded as a sacred herb.

Ruled by the Sun and the element Fire.

Therapeutic properties: Activates lethargic circulation during respiratory infections. Clears nasal passages during colds, bronchitis, or whooping cough.

Rosemary can be used in massage for rheumatism, gout, varicose veins and any condition due to poor circulation. Stimulates the scalp and helps reconstruct the damaged hair follicles; also useful for the digestive system, as it serves as a remedy for colitis and flatulence. Avoid in the first trimester of pregnancy.

Actions: Antispasmodic, carminative, cephalic, decongestant, digestive, stimulant, sudorific.

SAGE, CLARY
Salvia sclarea

Botanical family: Labiatae.

Principal components: Linalyl acetate, linalol, pinene, myrcene.

Climate of origin: Temperate dry, desert. Native to the Middle East and south of Europe.

Oil extracted from: Entire plant when flowering.

Produced in: Bulgaria, France, Morocco, Spain.

Blending class: Middle note.

Characteristics: A light greenish-yellow liquid with a pleasant herbal scent and mildly bitter taste; blends well with other herbal and citrus oils, and also with woods such as cedarwood and sandalwood.

History & lore: Another herb well-liked by the medieval herbalists and healers. The mucilaginous seeds were used for making a soothing slippery tea to wash and "clear" foreign bodies from the eyes. The name *clary* is thought to come from this fact. Clary sage has been known to have a narcotic-like effect, as documented by Robert Tisserand in *The Art of Aromatherapy*.

Widely used in the fragrance and food industry.

Ruled by the planet Mercury and the element Air.

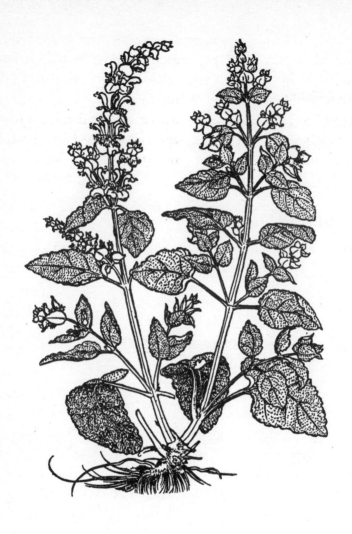

CLARY SAGE
Salvia sclarea

Therapeutic properties: Clary sage is both sedative and tonic, so think of clary when the condition is one of weakness coming from the nervous system and causing general physical debility or apathy. Good for use in any convalescent state. Rovesti and Gattefossé demonstrated in 1973 that it can lower high blood pressure. Clary sage has been used as a panacea since ancient times. Its high content of the component linalol qualifies it as an anesthetic.

I have successfully massaged diluted clary on the lower abdomen to diminish menstrual cramps. It has a wonderfully nurturing and soothing quality. It is a good companion for harmonization of the female cycle. Avoid in the first trimester of pregnancy.

Actions: Anesthetic, antidepressant, antispasmodic, hypotensor, sedative, tonic.

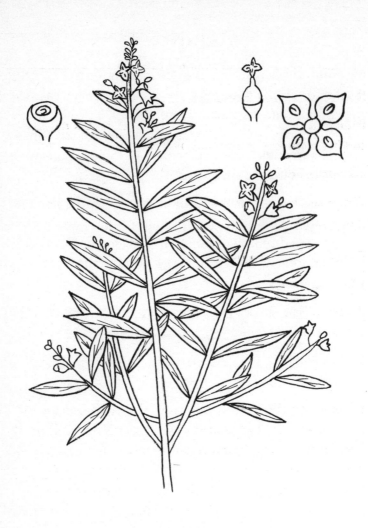

SANDALWOOD
Santalum album

Sandalwood
Santalum album

Botanical family: Santalaceae.

Principal components: Santalol, borneol, santalone, santine and other trace sesquiterpene hydrocarbons.

Climate of origin: Tropical. Native to Asia.

Produced in: India (Mysore), Indonesia and Taiwan.

Oil extracted from: Inner heartwood of large tree.

Produced in: India (Mysore), Indonesia, and Taiwan.

Blending class: Base note.

Characteristics: A heavy, viscous, clear-to-yellow oil with a wonderful sweet wood scent and a bitter, hot taste.

Blends well with most essential oils; the ones from herbs, as well as from resins and all floral oils.

History & lore: Sandalwood has been used for at least 4,000 years, and is often associated with meditation temples of the East. In India it is combined with rose oil to produce the famous perfume, aytar. In Asia, the wood is carved into scented boxes, furniture, and fine buildings. Sandalwood is used as an incense, as a main ingredient in the production of cosmetics, and for embalming. The oil is also used as a moisturizer for dry and rough skin.

Used by the fragrance industry as a fixative in high-class perfumery and cosmetics.

Ruled by the planet Uranus and the element Air.

Therapeutic properties: In Ayurvedic medicine sandalwood is used for treating urinary and respiratory infections, and diarrhea. In Chinese medicine it is a remedy for choleric intestines, stomach conditions, vomiting and gonorrhea.

Currently, sandalwood is used in English hospitals for the treatment of streptococcal throat infections.

Actions: Antiseptic, aphrodisiac, bactericidal, sedative, antiphlogistic, expectorant.

Tea Tree
Melaleuca alternifolia

Botanical family: Myrtaceae.

Principal components: Terpinene-4-ol, sesquiterpenes, cineol, pinene.

Climate of origin: Sub-tropical. Native to Australia.

Oil extracted from: Leaves and twigs of large tree.

Produced in: Australia.

Blending class: Middle note.

Characteristics: Light yellow or greenish oil with a very strong, balsamic/spicy, medicinal smell. It can yield a fresh note when blended with geranium, lavender or pine.

History & lore: Tea tree has been used in Australia for a long time, originally by the Aborigines. The name is attributed to the use of the leaves as a medicinal tea.

Therapeutic properties: Tea tree has antibacterial, antifungal and antiviral actions, thus serving as if it were many oils combined. Its most important therapeutic power is stimulation of the immune system.

Tea tree is a general antiseptic and cicatrisant, and is non-toxic. It can be used in any condition needing an anti-infectious action.

Actions: Antiseptic, antibacterial, antiviral, antifungal, immunostimulant, cicatrisant, expectorant, etc.

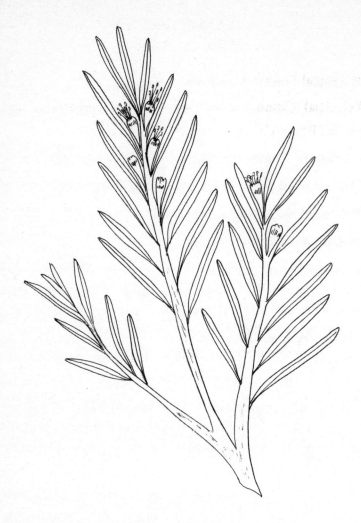

Tea Tree
Melaleuca alternifolia

YLANG YLANG
Cananga odorata

Botanical family: Anonaceae.

Principal Components: Linalol, farnesol, benzyl acetate, methyl para-cretol.

Climate of origin: Tropical. Native to Asia.

Oil extracted from: Flowers of large tree.

Produced in: Madagascar, Comoro Islands .

Blending Class: Base note.

Characteristics: Yellow in color, its scent is rather deep and strongly sweet. Serves well as a fixative in perfumery. Oil is produced with same flowers being distilled in successive distillations, First distillation is labeled as *extra*, then *second distillation*, third distillation, and *complete*, which is a mixture of all consecutive distillations.

History & lore: Widely used in perfumery as a floral, oriental note. It was used in Victorian Europe as a hair preparation. In Indonesia, where it grows, it is a tradition to cover a newly-wedded couple's bed with these strongly fragrant flowers. Oil is produced in different qualities.

Therapeutic Properties: An excellent medicine for anxiety and stress-related conditions, ylang ylang is a sexual tonic helpful for frigidity and impotence.

Actions: Anti-spasmodic, sexual stimulant, sedative.

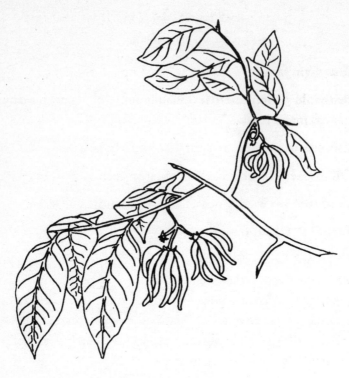

Ylang Ylang

Cananga odorata

Definitions of Therapeutic Actions

Analgesic: Eliminates pain.

Antidepressant: Uplifts negative states of mind.

Antiphlogistic: Constricts capillaries, leading to reduction of inflammation.

Antiseptic: Acts against the growth of bacteria.

Antispasmodic: Relaxes muscles suffering involuntary contractions.

Antitoxic: Acts against poisoning.

Aphrodisiac: Stimulates libido.

Astringent: Contracts tissues.

Carminative: Expels gas from intestines.

Cephalic: Relates to mental disorders, stimulates memory and sharpens focus.

Cicatrisant: Helps in the formation of scar tissue.

Cordial: Gives energy to the cardiac muscle, toning it.

Digestive: Promotes easy digestion.

Expectorant: Expels mucus from lungs, throat and sinus.

Galactagogue: Stimulates lactation.

Haemostatic: Stops bleeding, helps blood coagulation.

Hepatic: Gives energy to the liver, toning it.

Hypotensor: Lowers arterial blood pressure.

Rubefacient: Locally stimulates circulation, causing redness of skin.

Sedative: Calms the nervous system.

Stimulant: Speeds up metabolism.

Sudorific: Promotes or increases perspiration.

Tonic: Gives energy, invigorating the body, an organ or local tissue.

Uterine: Gives energy, toning to the uterus.

Vasoconstrictor: Constricts capillaries.

Vulnerary: Aids in healing external wounds.

Formulating with Essential Oils
Perfume Art

...The power of expression comes by getting into touch with the inner source from which these things come. A calm and silent mind is a great help for the free flow of the power.
~The Mother

The Egyptians related to perfume as a life-giving substance, and so deeply were they taken by the power of aromatic plants that one of their creation myths depicts an aromatic blue lotus flower as the first manifested form out of which their God Ra, the Sun, emerged. The Egyptians perfected techniques for extracting aromatic material from plants for use in cosmetics, medicine, and spiritual practices which utilized incense and perfumes.

Memphis hieroglyphs tell us of the God of perfume, Nefertum, who was associated with the aromatic lotus of creation. Nefertum, as *the soul of life*, would purify the body. (Van Toller and Dodd, Eds. *Fragrance: The Psychology and Biology of Perfume.*)

In modern times we have been so bombarded with sophisticated synthetic-aroma chemicals, that the confusion in our olfactory system often does not permit appreciation of pure blends containing oils from plant and flowers. As a civilization, how far we now find ourselves from the Egyptian way of honoring the Earth!

True botanical oils have a different "signatures"; they are much more vibrant and earthy in spite of their gentler interaction with the body. Modern-technology perfumes all use synthetic fixers—substances to keep aromatic molecules from evaporating quickly from the skin. Botanical perfumes interact with the skin, then naturally disappear into the environment, as if to remind us that their movement connects us to what lies beyond the physical world.

To a nose trained in botanical essential oils only, what is the aromatic message of the commercial perfume? Very simple, no mysteries:

"I am sophisticated, techno-smart, city inspired and concrete wise. I am here to stay on your skin through sweat and showers for at least 36 hours. In your heart, I constantly hook you up to the high caste of society. In your mind I constantly remind you of the fashion models I am associated with, between the strips in the magazines…You can become me…through me, you will be like a million other identity seekers, unwavering believers…Little do you know how I can hide your true identity. I can rescue you from human odor and give you a sexy cross between a bon-bon and a space shuttle lubricant with a few faux flowers sprinkled over it."

Perhaps this assessment is being a little ungrateful to the tremendous scientific efforts to lift us off the ground, but when the mind transcends science and modern ideas become passé, spirit always remains.

Spirit is what I like to call the dynamics of botanical essence— something that moves and changes like life does. That which holds the mystery of crossing the doorway into the invisible dimensions of existence.

I love to remember my own smell. It tells me a lot about who I am.

When I spread a pure flower essence on my skin, I think about that flower and her world. When the scent disappears, does it go back into the dimension of flower consciousness? When my own body smell merges with the scent of a flower, I am clearly aware of an interactive natural synergy.

Aromatherapists and botanical perfumers seek knowledge, knowledge about our relationship with the plant world. It is exciting to think of becoming aware of the vibrational codes coming from a plant whispering messages about life on earth.

Blending Essential Oils

When you blend essential oils, you are working with the visible oils and their physical properties, and the invisible element of their smells, which will serve you as a guide.

There are some common-sense facts about blending that we will begin to explore in this book, but there is also a level of learning about blending that relies on one's experience and intuition. Experience can only come with time, and in this art, it comes with smelling, blending, applying and observing; so if you are interested in aromatherapy, you ought to start and *keep smelling* essential oils as often as possible. This will naturally make memory records for the smells. Soon you will be gathering experience and feeling more and more confident in what you are doing with the oils.

Intuition is very important in blending, and I believe intuition can be invoked if the right state of mind is exercised. We all have the same potential, but this potential needs to be activated in order to function. Sometimes I think about blending in the same way I think about cooking: it's an alchemical process that needs more than what you do with your hands and a recipe to turn out great. What is in the mind matters, and the motivation and intention is principal. I tell my students that the most important intention to begin with is to create a harmonious blend, and you do this by having a harmonious mind as you work, holding the feeling of believing in the abilities of the self. Choose to create something simple, and don't mix more than three oils to start. Take the three oils and learn about them first. There is so much to learn about how concentrations work in blending, even with just two oils! Safe choices for blending are oils that contain the same components. (See previous Essential Oils pages.)

Oils have a character depending on their composition, the climate they grew in, the altitude at which they grew, and the soil, just to mention a few factors. Since essential oils have therapeutic properties, I find it easy to equate their characters with their healing functions.

Surely plants assist human beings on all levels: physical, emotional, mental and spiritual. This is an important reason to think of your blend holistically. When you are blending oils for a formula, this formula ideally should address body, mind, spirit and emotion. Your work becomes the art of putting together something synergistic, not only because the smell of each oil must enhance the others in the blending to create a greater sum than the separate parts combined (the concept of synergy), but also the separate therapeutic properties must synergize to bring a total harmony of body, mind, spirit and emotion. Consider the holistic need of the person you do aromatherapy for, before you focus your intention on the search for an end result.

Next, you must know how to dilute oils in the right proportions. You will be using mostly vegetable oils as carriers of your essential oils. Essential oils do not go rancid, but vegetable oils do, so you will have to add vitamin E to your blend as a natural preservative. You can also blend essential oils with alcohol or vinegar.

Following is a list of vegetable oils you can use:

Almond oil: Sweet and fine, but I find it the most fragile oil in terms of spoiling. Use with a few capsules of vitamin E, and blend small quantities at a time.

Avocado oil: Vitamin-rich, highly nutritious oil, good to carry facial oil blends for dry and depleted skins. Fairly resistant to spoilage.

Grapeseed oil: Grapeseed is a lot like almond oil, but it has a natural vitamin E content, making it more resistant to oxidation or rancidity. It is all-purpose and good for massage blends.

Hazelnut oil: Fine and luxurious, with a sweet aroma. Use with a few capsules of vitamin E.

Jojoba oil: Actually a liquid wax and not an oil. Carrier for perfume blend concentrations. Does not oxidize.

Sesame oil: Wonderful, even plain, for a sun lotion; it has a mild natural sunscreen. Add a few capsules of vitamin E.

I like to use the less-common rice bran and aloe vera oils in face and baby oils, for their extremely fine texture. It is good to blend them with a small amount of a more nutritious oil, such as the vegetable nut oils listed above.

About Your Blend Concentration

Keep in mind that the concentration of aromatic composition inside the living plant is usually between 3 percent to 10 percent. One may create *concentrate* blends to be extended later. Perfumes can be *extracts*, up to 35 percent essential oils and absolutes. I recommend that beginners use low concentrations in their blends, to understand how therapeutically powerful they can be. (Molecules in dispersion go through the layers of skin much more easily.) Using low concentrations will also be safer and help train the sense of smell.

The measurements given below will vary depending on the density of each oil and size of the drop applicator. The denser the oil, the fewer drops you will need.

1 ounce = approximately 30 ml (29.57ml).
10 percent of one ounce = approximately 60 to 90 drops.
1 milliliter = 20 to 35 drops.
1 drop = 0.03 ml.

Following are basic guidelines for average concentrations:

Bath: 5 to 15 drops per bath.
Massage oil: 10 to 15 drops per ounce.
Lotion: 15 drops per ounce.
Facial oil: 6 to 12 drops per ounce.
Facial clay: 3 to 5 drops per ounce.
Hair treatment oil: 20 drops per ounce.
Fragrance: 10 percent to 45 percent, depending on density and odor intensity.

The Art of Making Perfumes

When blending oils to create a perfume, think of smells as you would colors: there is no guarantee that two pretty colors will look prettier after you have mixed them. The aspect that you have to work with, besides your intuition and experience, is chemical compatibility. (For component listing see previous Essential Oils pages.)

Odor intensity is important because one oil can completely overpower another. Take pieces of blotter or acid-free watercolor paper and pour one drop of each oil you want to blend, separately. Notice, and maybe even time, how long it takes for each smell to go away. This will give you a pretty good idea of odor intensity. The most persistent scents should be used a lot less in your blend than the ones that are mild-smelling and disappear faster. This brings us to the classification of oils for blending, usually referred to as base, middle and top notes.

Base notes are the wise old folks who are calmer, slower, and most times physically denser. Think of them as the hard drive of a computer which has memory to store outside information. They are the fixers of botanical perfumery; less volatile, and can keep other oils in the blend from evaporating too quickly.

Middle notes: These are the oils that can be used more generously in a blend because they are the mildest smells, the ones that "round the corners," meaning that they help equalize oppositions. They are smell mediators, acting as the diplomats of a composition, negotiating chemical balances and smoothing out differences. They are the hardest oils to detect in the finished blend, as they tend to do their job and "integrate," becoming invisible. One can sense their work, but can't remember their personality as easily as with the other oils.

Top notes: These are the flamboyant, bombastic, young and restless bunch. They have to make a quick and strong presence, and then disappear so you can't catch them. They are important because they add that unforgettable spark to the blend, making it interesting. Be careful with them, as they are sharp, penetrating, and very volatile and likely will be the ones to give you the most trouble.

Although the perfume industry has a standard classification for the perfume notes category, here is my own classification of the oils included in this book that are aesthetically pleasing for perfume making:

Base notes: Frankincense, jasmine, rose, sandalwood, ylang ylang.

Middle notes: Bergamot, geranium, lemon, neroli, clary sage.

Top notes: Basil, chamomile, lavender, peppermint, rosemary.

Perfume Signatures & The Esscènt™ Method

Essential oil synergy is the creation of a biodynamic mixture, which reveals a chemically complex composition resulting in the living energy field of an aromatic formula. What I am speaking of can be a formulation to scent a product, or a perfume.

If you mix one drop of orange oil with one drop of lavender, it will not be considered a synergy. In this case each oil alone would have a powerful influence. However, if to six drops of orange is added two drops of lavender, a synergistic effect could result. Why? Consider sprinkling cinnamon on applesauce or adding a bright-colored detail to a neutral-color dress. The effect should create something that feels complete in itself, a unit of something original. Each oil has a specific amount to offer to the composition, which forms the aromatic relationship. Sometimes one particular oil adds more to the whole than another. Considerations of odor intensity, evaporation rates and density need to be well thought out.

This knowledge is also learned intuitively as one experiences essential oil blending. It can become quite complex and challenging, the more one ventures into the relationships of oils. Intuition plays a role that can translate into numbers or parts, drops or liquid measurements.

I discovered in my early blending experiments that oils from different plant parts required different proportions for a successful synergy. Essential oils are sometimes distilled from the entire plant, as in the case of most herbal oils, but many others are distilled from a single plant part, be the fruit rind or resin, root, wood trunk or leaves, the flower or the seed of a plant.

In 1984, I experienced for the first time the desire to help people with my discovery of a therapy using scent from true plant oils to modify the emotional and mental state of someone in crisis, or going through a stressful time. This also can help people link up to a natural support system through the most powerful and intriguing sensual language, smell.

This was the beginning of my path in the exciting new field of aromatherapy. I became aware of the potential that perfumes made from natural and pure plant-source oils have in therapy, because these oils have therapeutic properties and can be safely inhaled deeply.

Now imagine that as a small child, while strolling in a lavender field you were stung by a bee, causing tremendous distress. Lavender has the therapeutic property to sedate the nervous system, but for you, who will have the association of a stressful experience, the smell of lavender oil will not serve as a sedative. This is a simple illustration to explain the complexity of using smell as therapy. So how is a therapist going to know how to blend an aromatic composition for a client? Is it going to work?

Looking for a solution, I created a method performed as psychotherapy using aroma, today known in my practice as the Esscènt sessions. I gather the client's smell preferences, the positive associations, in order to blend a custom formulation that serves as a tool in this smell therapy. This perfume contains the best smell associations chosen by the client, going through the different plant parts: roots, resin, wood, leaf, branch, fruit, flower and seed. The specific aromatic molecules that make up the composition, the personal aromatic signature, feeds into the individual's energy field, transmitting well-being to positively affect body, mind and emotion. This is one of the vibrational healing modalities—psychotherapy using aroma.

A new smell, experienced for the first time, holds tremendous potential for a conscious association to be made with a therapeutic purpose. In my work in the Esscènt sessions, I lead the client with imagery in order to reprogram negative mental patterns into new, positive ones, using the smell to create a memory record for this new association.

After all these years and many, many sessions of making therapeutic perfumes, I have now the experience to say that people can access emotional healing and mental harmony by using a personal *therapeutic perfume*, one that contains all of their best memories with favorable emotional content. This is my story of how I began to make perfumes—by making personalized formulas using this method I created for clients whom I considered "patients."

My Esscènt sessions are divided into two separate personal meetings where a total of thirty essential oils and absolutes are smelled and screened by the participant. This method uses a kit containing aromas in a set of vials, into which I place small pieces of blotter paper containing a drop or two of each essential oil, and a chart to note down the preferences. The different smells are screened from -2 for a sure rejection, -1 for a dislike, 0 for a feeling of neutrality, +1 for a positive reaction and +2 for a definite preference. After creating this chart by smelling the aromas, the client turns the scores over to me. Then I take this numeric information to my lab to create the perfume according to the preferences of the client, arranging the right balance between base, middle and top notes.

I find this to be a unique method, not only because it is positively empowering to an individual to have their own signature perfume made with their best smell associations, using therapeutic oils that are safe to inhale, but also because it is a process done consciously, and with the client's input for a therapeutic result. I have learned so much about people's personalities and their problems, what seems to empower them and how all this relates to the smell preferences for the different oils, in a perspective of psycho-aromatherapy. When I am blending a personal perfume for someone, I feel that person telling me how to compose a certain harmony having to do with the very best of themselves, then put that message in a bottle.

The Creation Story of a Perfume

Invisible and fragrant… a volatile composition evaporates into the air, and is inhaled. Smell sensations are processed in the brain, and stimulate emotional responses.

It's late summer. I am in my lab at 6:55 am, ready to continue writing my ideas on therapeutic perfumes. I am holding my inner sense of fullness with specific information, and feeling the importance of sharing this material with others. But I feel torn between writing and blending perfume. On my clipboard are the results from my last Esscènt session with a sweet and sensual, fun-loving young woman. For privacy, here I will call her simply SHE, the word we women sometimes use to define the Goddess.

I ponder over her therapeutic perfume, her aromatic signature to be. As she merges with it, SHE will remember her own essence, her truth, and her power. It crosses my mind that receiving this new scent at this time in her life will undoubtedly support her with the emotional turmoil that she is feeling. Smell and emotion. They are forever inseparable in our minds, in ways that we may never even faintly suspect.

I begin to pull down from my shelves all the essential oils and extracts in her preference list. Now I focus on her soul. At the same time, I am making these notes, and including her as my secret character in this story, as I begin her perfume creation.

I am remembering her session, and look at my notes. SHE loves people, world cultures, and music. Mental confusion makes her irrational and severely frustrated. I call upon her higher self, her personal angel on duty. I feel it with me here.

As SHE experienced one neutral (zero) preference, she had a comment, "This smell is intriguing, maybe I should say a zero with an opening to a +1." I open a bottle with this smell and take a sniff: ahhh… *Boswellia carterii*, frankincense. I had learned previously that frankincense has an ability to sweeten citrus smells, so I look for the citrus oils in her file, and notice that three out of four citrus smells are in her maximum preferences. Frankincense is a resin, considered by me in a general way as a representative of the innermost essence of self. The idea comes to blend it with citrus oils, fruit rinds, which I understand as representing that part in us that opens, and can be nurturing, nourishing aspects of life. This seems to fit as a solid piece in the puzzle I am putting together for her fragrant creation that will be the living symbol of her wholeness.

Roses. SHE must have roses. SHE grades highly both *Damascena otto* and *Rose maroc* absolute, as well as geranium. Geranium is a kindred composition to rose, and will strengthen the power of the alcohol geraniol in the formula; all three oils have geraniol as a noble component. Geraniol will bring a tough sweetness, like the skin of young native girls. Yes! resin and fruit mixed with roses—I feel a decisive moment. My character as creative detective is once again manifested in full regalia at this point. I am on. SHE has gotten me engaged in my creative center to manifest her therapeutic perfume to perfection.

Now for the rose mathematics, measurements relating to smell. Bringing the first one to the nose, *Rosa damascena*:

strong, unique, noble. Second, geranium: strong but specific, very present. Third, *Rosa centifolia*; sweet, soft, warm, gentle, and welcoming. Numbers pour into my mind: one drop of *Rosa damascena*, two drops of geranium, and four drops of *Rosa centifolia*. Mixing geranium with Damasc rose gives it a "growing with knowledge" feeling, like learning something important from your own grandmother.

I am thinking, why is it so obvious to me that aromatic compositions mean information? Rose has a much more complex existence than geranium, but as kindred compositions one can enhance the other in a way of growth, integrating their information into a larger body of knowledge. Next I pour in four drops of *Rosa centifolia* and mix vigorously, lab style, clasping the tube at the top lip with left hand and shaking between pointy and middle finger of right hand. Taking in the smell; geranium is too present. I need another hundred roses (two drops), or to start over with less. I am so glad that the Esscènt perfume is not constricted by price; this is a free-flowing moment of alchemical magic. I decide to start over. Later, with seven precious drops of rose and geranium I will make myself a luxurious gift of rose massage oil.

One drop of geranium, one of *Rosa damascena* and four of *Rosa centifolia*, perfect. Now I have the rose segment blend for her formula. Next is frankincense. Mysterious, and yes, intriguing, as SHE said. For all of that, only half of a drop goes into the mixture. *Jasmine sambac*, for it is closer to orange blossom absolute in smell because of the component neroliol: one drop…here is the base note. Creating a harmonious blend of citrus oils in nearly equal measure makes a smooth body for the formula: eight grapefruit, eight bergamot, four lemon, and two petitgrain for a more "raw nature" feel. Frankincense, with many times less the evaporation rate of volatile citrus essence, seems to slow down the speedy feel of citrus oils. Into the rose base this goes…oh fresh!

Now for the top note. The element of excitement. I want to give her the spices of her choice. I feel her angel nodding its head at me. Sweet spice of nutmeg and cardamom is delicious, but I know I have to go gingerly with it. The sensuality of jasmine needs to be close to the healing strength of clary sage, one not to be forgotten from her preferences. Meandering with the spicy notes of cardamom and nutmeg will give the richness of her soul a stroke, I am sure. This is hardly a top note at all; it is the presence of overwhelming delight unobstructed by rules.

Again, the smell math. Clary sage and nutmeg are so harmonious together, wishing to go side by side; I give one drop of each. Cardamom speaks louder, but I just want to give it the same importance, so I must raise the numbers of the former to two each; two drops of nutmeg, two of clary, and one of cardamom. Coming to a close, I must check all the other numbers in the formula and take note of this final spice decision. This is one of those perfumes where segments are worked out as if separate formulas, to be blended together for a final equation. Yes, it is fine! The wonderful action of a citrus influence is that it can "wrap up" a complex formula such as this one, but with care, in the right measure, not to lessen the precious drops of flowers.

Now with all the twelve densities of oils in the completed formula, I have precisely one milliliter. I am extending it with jojoba to make a five-milliliter perfume extract vial, so the perfume composition contains one fifth raw plant material, twenty percent of the total blend. I shake this vigorously, and put it to rest for the night.

Now it's the morning after. Excitedly I take in the smell again, do my lab shake one more time, and begin to pour more jojoba oil into the fragrant composition. I go one milliliter at a time, shaking, smelling, and noticing the changes in my freshly-made batch of fragrant fluid. It is fascinating to observe its biodynamic character changing as the scent moves across its dilution.

Beauty / Cosmetic Aromatherapy

What is holistic about aromatherapy skin care?

> Nourishment for the skin.
> Healing for the soul.
> Relaxation for the mind.

Do it yourself for self-empowerment and creative stimulation.

Thee three levels cited above are connected. The skin, being the outer and largest organ of the body, is the best representation of the overall health of the body. The harmonious balance of all parts of the individual—the body, the emotions and the mind—represents the health condition of the body. Where one is at risk of being out of balance, so are all the other connecting parts. The use of essential oils on the skin is also the use of essential oils on the emotions and mind. The differences in skin type are also differences in the emotional and mental makeup of each individual. So, fine aromatherapy skin care, by conscious intent, will address all aspects of an individual. Ideally, one practicing aromatherapy will make personalized skin care treatments.

I am an advocate of kitchen cosmetics. They may not be as easy to apply, or have a long shelf life or the fantastic claims that the sophisticated new-technology cosmetics do, but the benefits of fresh food for your skin, and the personal creative involvement which gives you emotional empowerment in your skin care (which is also very economical), by far surpasses the benefit of commodity, in my opinion.

Cosmetic and companies rely on the sensational advertisement of the use of some of the same ingredients in their formulas. Why not use these ingredients while they are pure and unprocessed, containing their maximum amount of vital energy, and know exactly what you are putting on your skin?

The knowledge that I am sharing with you in the following pages has come from my common sense; trial-and-error experimentations; intuition; and constant reading to evaluate books and articles on nutrition, herbalism, beauty, and aromatherapy. I have had wonderful teachers such as Rosemary Gladstar and Dr. Kurt Schnaubelt of the Pacific Institute of Aromatherapy, who gave me a terrific start. I have had a life-long practice of creating experiments and observing different treatments on my and other's skins. Before my aromatherapy practice, I had already been using herbs and food for beauty, and with the addition of essential oils, the pleasure and good results have been multiplying!

In 1986, when I worked in the spas in the hot springs resorts of Calistoga, California, as a massage therapist and facialist, I devised a basic natural skin care system using fresh food materials and essential oils. Ever since that time this system has been evolving to accommodate my skin's changing needs and those of friends and family, which covers from teen to mature skins.

Skin Care

My system consists of preparations to address the following functions of skin care: To clean, to moisturize, to nourish, to stimulate and to heal.

To clean: Use the scrubs as a soap or cleanser substitute to wash the dead cells off the skin surface daily. Use clay masks for deep pore cleansing once a week.

To moisturize: You need water and oil; use this combination in a homemade cream or milk. If you are a purist, try the same combination in separate steps: First use a wrung-out steaming hot wash cloth, cover face for a minute to open pores, then spray floral waters or pat with lukewarm herbal tea, following with aromatherapy facial oils, massaging face in gentle upward circular strokes until the water and the oils are absorbed; or you can steam face, then apply oils. The easiest way is to use facial oils immediately after showering when skin is saturated with water and pores are open. Oily skin does not need daily creams or facial oils; use herbal steams and honey masks with essential oils instead.

To nourish: Use masks made from fresh food containing vitamins, proteins and minerals; use fruit, nut butters, seaweed, yeast, algae, honey, and herbs. Only apply nourishing masks after skin cleansing.

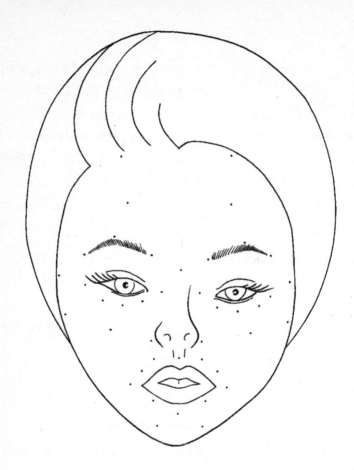

Acupressure Points.

To stimulate: Use temperature changes to contract and expand blood vessels, causing an increase in blood circulation. Alternate hot and cold with a washcloth or steam face, then apply herbal cold splash or rosemary water spray; follow with acupressure points. (See opposite page.)

For facials, contract blood vessels using clay or astringent herbs, egg whites and essential oils; expand with steam and calming facial oils.

Stimulate skin when it is sluggish, dull or discolored.

To heal: Use essential oil blends with carrier oils or nut milks, herbs, honey and vitamin E. Heal skin when it has acne, is irritated, inflamed or blemished.

The **Basic Skin Care** is to clean and moisturize once or twice a day; deep pore cleansing and nourishing once a week.

The **Complete Facial**, done once a month, in the following order of application, consists of these steps:

The scrub, to prepare skin surface for facial.

A clay mask for deep pore cleansing (use clay of your choice and mix with enough water to make a smooth cream. Add 4 to 6 drops of essential oils, according to skin type, and keep mixing into the smooth cream). Let mask dry completely before the herbal steam.

To do an herbal steam, place a handful of herbs in a bowl and cover the herbs with half a bowl of boiling water, then cover bowl with a bath towel for a few seconds; close your eyes and slide your face into the steam just above the bowl with the towel sealed around your head. Stay under the towel until steam cools down. You can blow on the water to speed the rising of steam. You can also use essential oils in the water. In this case, only a drop or less of oils, and stir the water.

After steaming, wipe off clay with a steaming hot, wrung-out washcloth until clay is completely removed, using gentle, circular, upward strokes. Rinse with lukewarm water. Now your pores are deeply clean and ready to absorb the vital fresh food in nourishing masks. (Recipes follow).

Moisturize skin with a combination of facial oils and herbal or floral water spray, facial cream or milk.

The final step in this routine is to stimulate acupressure points and splash with cold herbal tea or spray with hydrolates. Allow skin to air dry.

The following recipes are some of what I have tested and reworked for the last twenty years. The ingredients described on the following pages are to be applied in the recipes, which are a sample set of simple as well as more complex formulas for daily use and for aromatherapy facials. These illustrate some of the results we can obtain with homemade cosmetics once we like to experiment with doing it ourselves. Study this information, try mixing some of these formulas and then create your own!

Before choosing a recipe or an ingredient for mixing your own preparation, determine the skin type you are working with. Dry skin feels taut. Normal skin feels smooth and supple. Oily skin feels greasy all over, sometimes with pimples and acne. Mixed skin is normal skin with shiny/oily areas such as nose and chin. Treat mixed skin as separate parts; treat oily areas with applications for oily skin and treat remaining areas with applications for normal skin. Sensitive skin develops rashes easily and is delicate. Inflamed skin has acne, redness, and abrasion.

Ingredient Descriptions

Following are some of the alive and edible elements of the homemade skin care recipes in this book, all available in good health food stores.

Almonds: Alkaline food rich in calcium/magnesium, protein and fat. Can be used on the skin as a milk, butter or pulp mixed with essential oils. Buy organic nuts.

Almond milk recipe: To produce one cup of almond milk, soak 20 medium- to large-size almonds in drinking water overnight, or pour boiling water over almonds and let it sit for 30 minutes. (This method is the easiest to peel almonds prior to blending if so desired.) Next, drain the water and put almonds in a cup of fresh water to whiz on high speed in a blender for 2 minutes or until a smooth, creamy consistency. Squeeze pulp through a fine sieve or through a cotton cloth bag (the gold coffee strainers work great); now you have the precious milk! If you don't use immediately, refrigerate, as it is energy-packed and highly perishable. It will last about three days if refrigerated.

The remaining solid mass is the pulp that can be used in scrubs for face and body. You can make a powder by drying the pulp in a low oven and pulverizing in a grinder. It is great for scrubs, especially mixed with honey. For sensitive skin I recommend peeling the almonds before blending. This may be quite a bit of work, but I guarantee the results will give you a purer quality and yield more milk! All skin types.

Aloe Vera: This is a mucilaginous plant. Use gel or juice; cooling, soothing and healing to skin abrasion, rashes, burns. If you have a plant, open the succulent leaf and use the gel inside; or you can buy aloe vera juice bottled with at least 95 percent pure juice.

Black Currant Seed Oil: Contains fatty acids high in gamma-linoleic acid, a substance that supports the reconstruction of damaged skin and other cell membranes. Good to add to healing formulas for acne and inflamed skins. Use combined with Vitamin E, and mix small quantities at a time. Keep refrigerated to avoid rancidity.

Borage Oil: Has the same property described above for black currant seed oil; keep refrigerated.

Brewers Yeast: Microscopic plant called *Saccharomyces Cerevisiae*. It is a food powder or flakes containing the entire B vitamin complex and concentrated protein with all amino acids. Nutrient. All skin types.

Clay: Deep cleanser of the pores; all clays have negative ionic charge. It pulls harmful positive ions from the toxins being eliminated by the skin. Absorbs debris and oil, which is washed off the skin with the clay after it dries. When mixed in water, clays have a drawing action as they dry, from their high swelling and shrinking factor, making skin contract. Clays occur under or on the ground all around the world; they can have different colors according to their mineral content; some are iron rich, the red, brown and black ones; some are copper-rich, the green ones; some are cobalt-rich, the blue ones, which are cooling and good to use in inflamed skin conditions; some are pure white. All have drawing and drying action, some more than others. After clay therapy, always moisturize the skin.

Bentonite is the most drawing clay; recommended for oily skin, as it easily absorbs excess oil on the skin. Unfortunately it is the most difficult clay to mix and to wash off.

Kaolin is my favorite clay. It is an easy to mix, all-purpose, hydrous aluminum silicate. It is creamy, fine white clay used in making porcelain. It is perfect for normal, dry, and sensitive skin for its smooth, clean and gentle drawing feel. It's very versatile and it lends itself well to mixing with any textured ingredient, such as sticky honey or fibrous fruit pulp.

Comfrey: A very healing, mucilaginous herb. The root has a high content of allantoin, a substance that supports the building of new cells. Dry or fresh leaves can be used in facial steams and powdered leaves can be used as healing poultices mixed with honey. Skin type: inflamed/acne.

Enzymes: Needed for all processes of metabolism. Anti-oxidant agents and catalysts aid other cells in eliminating, coagulating, building cells and decomposing. Enzymes attack waste material and can help protect the skin against harmful bacteria. Use an enzyme-rich liquid for mixing into facial masks or as a digestive drink.

Rejuvelac Recipe: Soak organic grains such as wheat, or dried fruits, in at least twice the volume of spring water at warm temperature, until tiny bubbles form and float to surface (24 hours). Drain and refrigerate. It will keep for many weeks, and will smell foul when too old.

Evening Primrose Oil: Skin cell restoration aid. Highest percentage of gamma-linoleic acid, which supports the reconstruction of damaged cell membranes. It has a therapeutic action on many of the body systems such as circulatory, digestive and the neuro-endocrine complex. Keep refrigerated. All skin types.

Honey: Natural bactericide; helps equalize ph acid/alkaline balance on the skin. Can be used as a cleanser, especially on oily skin when no oil or milks are desired. Honey is also an emollient, softening agent, full of life force, energizing to the skin as it creates the perfect base for powdered herbs and foodstuffs in scrubs. Use unprocessed honey. Soap substitute. All skin types.

Hydrolates: Also known as hydrosols or floral water sprays, this is the water resulting from the condensation of steam distillation after the essential oils have been removed. Hydrosols are saturated with hydrophilic compounds which are present in plants, but not in the essential oils. These compounds are water-soluble. They include the carboxylic acids that are the most calming therapeutic elements found in plants. Harsh compounds, such as aggressive terpene hydrocarbon alcohols found in essential oils, are dissolved in the hydrosols due to their hydroxyl group. Beneficial properties of terpene and sesquiterpene alcohols include antiseptics, lymphatic decongestants, tonics and stimulants.

Hydrolates are completely safe for all skins, especially eye care applications, including inflamed and infected conditions. Chamomile is the mildest, rose is the most astringent and neroli the most hydrating. Lavender can be considered the most all-purpose.

Nut Butters: These nutrients can also work as emollients for the skin, containing protein, fat, and important minerals such as calcium, a nerve-ending tranquilizer; magnesium, which helps absorption of calcium and activates some enzymes; and iron. Choose from almond, Brazil nut, cashews, macadamia, and vitamin E-rich sesame seed butter, or tahini. Always mix with honey. All skin types.

Rose Hip Seed Oil: Also known as *Rosa rubiginosa* or *Rosa mosqueta*, it is an important oil from the seed of a South American variety of the wild rose. Similar to evening primrose oil, very rich in gammalinoleic acid; prevents skin cell membrane damage. All skin types, particularly useful for skin affected by premature aging.

Seaweed: Edible sea vegetable with a high concentration of minerals that are important in skin care. Rich in iodine which stimulates circulation, calcium for reducing nerve-ending irritability, and iron for toning facial muscles. Kelp powder and dulse flakes are best suited for skin use. All skin types.

Slippery Elm: An herbal powder with mucilaginous properties. Softens and helps soothe inflammation and infections of the mucus membranes. A protective agent. It is good mixed with fibrous materials such as powdered dry herbs in scrubs. Skin types: dry, sensitive, and inflamed/acne.

Spirulina: Anti-oxidant. Green algae in powder form. It is a concentrated food containing chlorophyll, a blood purifier. Contains 60 percent protein; vitamin A, which protects the skin from infection; and all the B vitamins, the vitamins with the most important organic functions for the skin. Very powerful nutrient for facial masks. All skin types.

Vitamin E: Anti-oxidant. Helps eradicate free radicals, those unbalanced molecules containing unpaired electrons that seek for their electrons in cell membranes and body-building proteins, causing alterations in molecular structure and creating an unbalanced chain reaction. Vitamin E can be used in homemade cosmetics as a natural preservative. All skin types.

ESSENTIAL OILS AND SKIN TYPES

Normal skin: Chamomile (blue and Roman), clary sage, geranium, lavender, neroli, rose, sandalwood.

Oily skin: Clary sage, eucalyptus, lavender, lemon, peppermint, rose, rosemary, and tea tree.

Dry/sensitive skin: Chamomile (blue and Roman), frankincense, lavender, neroli.

Inflamed/acne: Chamomile (blue and Roman), clary sage, lavender, lemon, neroli, tea tree.

Mature skin: Clary sage, frankincense, lavender, neroli, rose, sandalwood.

HERBS AND SKIN TYPES

Use these in steams and powder them for scrubs.

Normal skin: Chamomile, lavender, peppermint, rose.

Oily skin: Lavender, peppermint, rose, rosemary, sage.

Dry/sensitive skin: Basil, chamomile, comfrey, lavender, mullein.

Acne/Inflamed skin: Chamomile, comfrey, lavender, mullein, rose.

Fruit and Skin Care

Many fruits have special nutritional values for making nourishing skin applications.

Cucumber: Botanically a fruit, it is an astringent with a toning quality. Contains protein and digestive enzymes. Rich in vitamins A, C and calcium.

Honeydew melon: Skin cleanser rich in vitamins A and C. Can be a substitute for papaya and strawberries in some formulas. Dry skin.

Papaya: Helps activate blood circulation in the capillaries. Contains the enzyme papain, which breaks down protein for better absorption. Contains vitamins A and C. It is a luxurious emollient, softening skin as it nourishes.

Pineapple: Enzyme-rich juice containing vitamins A and C. Helps sluggish skin activate blood circulation in the capillaries.

Strawberry: Skin cleanser rich in vitamins A and C. Helps skin to eliminate toxins. Pulp has been traditionally used as poultices to alleviate sore eyes.

Tomato: Natural antiseptic. Purifying agent rich in vitamins A and C, calcium/magnesium. Good for skin blemishes, pimples and acne.

Exotic Kitchen Recipes

Recipe for almond milk and rejuvelac can be found on Ingredient Descriptions, pages 111 and 113.

Notes: *Tanacetum Annuum* is a wonderful oil containing azulene components, which I like to use as an alternative to blue chamomile in these formulas. The scent is much more desirable than the common German or "blue" chamomile.

The rosemary that I use, which is more appropriate for skin care, is chemotype *Rosemary verbanon*. See Appendix for sources of oils you can't find at a store near you.

The Scrubs

Scrubs are soap and cleanser substitutes for daily use prior to moisturizing the skin. Apply on wet skin, but avoid getting water in the scrub jar. These scrubs are fairly stable, but best kept away from heat and direct sunlight. These recipes make approximately 1 ounce.

Simple scrub for all skin types

2 T of brewers yeast
2 T of raw honey
Essential oil:
6 drops of lavender oil
Mix lavender oil into honey; stir in yeast until smooth.

Fancy scrub for normal skin

2 T of dried rose petals
1 T of dried lavender flowers
1 chamomile tea bag
6 macadamia nuts
honey
Essential oils:
3 drops of Roman chamomile
2 drops of lavender
2 drops of clary sage
1 drop of neroli

You will need a mortar and pestle and a clean coffee or nut grinder or similar implement.

Grind your rose petals to smaller flakes. Grind nuts into fine meal in mortar.

Add essential oils to nut meal and mix. Add nut meal and lavender flowers to grinder and run it a few times with the ground rose petals until mixture resembles an even fine meal; be careful not to overdo it.

Mix chamomile petals from tea bag into the rest of the mix. Save this mix and prepare one ounce at a time with equal parts of honey for your daily use. Use ¼ ounce mix and ¼ ounce honey. Apply the scrub on wet face with gentle circular, upward strokes and rinse with lukewarm water.

Simple scrub for oily skin

    1 teaspoon of sesame butter (tahini)
    1 tablespoon of raw honey
    1 teaspoon of brewer's yeast
    1 teaspoon of kelp granules or powder
    Essential oils:
    1 drop of peppermint
    3 drops of lavender
    6 drops of lemon

Pour essential oils into honey and mix well. Add tahini. Mix in dry ingredients last, one at a time, mixing vigorously until smooth. It should have a stiff consistency. Spread it on wet face in circular, upward strokes. Wash off with lukewarm water and a final cold splash.

Simple scrub for normal to oily skin with acne and pimples

    2 chamomile tea bags
    2 tablespoons of honey
    Essential oils:
    1 drop of blue chamomile
    2 drops of Roman chamomile
    1 drop of lavender

Mix essential oils into a 1-ounce glass jar then pour honey into jar, mixing with the oils. Pour contents of tea bags into honey/essential oils mixture and mix until smooth. Apply with gentle circular upward strokes on wet face and rinse with lukewarm water.

Fancy scrub for inflamed/acne

1 T of fresh almond meal (resulting from preparation of almond milk, see recipe on page 111)
1 T of aloe vera juice
1 T of comfrey powder
1 T of mullein powder
1 T of honey
Essential oils:
6 drops of lemon
4 drops of tea tree
2 drops of rosemary verbanon

Powder herbs in grinder, then push through a tea strainer to remove the larger bits. Mix essential oils into honey. Mix all wet ingredients, and add powder. Apply to dry skin with gentle circular upward stokes. Rinse with lukewarm water. It will keep for three days if refrigerated.

THE FACIAL OILS

The following formulas will make 15 milliliters of facial oil.

15 milliliters = 1 tablespoon = 300 drops

For each recipe, mix essential oils first in a small glass bottle, then pour in the other oils and shake. It will not go rancid if you keep it in a cool, dark place. Use after a scrub, shower, steam or herbal/floral/spray. See Appendix for material sources.

Normal skin:

5 milliliters of hazelnut or grapeseed oil
8 milliliters of rice bran oil
2 capsules of evening primrose oil
2 capsules of Vitamin E
Essential oils:
2 drops of frankincense
2 drops of rose otto
1 drop of neroli
1 drop of Roman chamomile

Dry/sensitive skin:

8 milliliters of aloe vera oil
5 milliliters of avocado oil
1 milliliters of rose hip oil
1 capsule of vitamin E
Essential oils:
1 drop of lavender
2 drops of Roman chamomile
1 drop of blue chamomile
4 drops of sandalwood

The Milks

See recipe for making fresh almond milk under Ingredient-Descriptions. Refrigerated, milks last a few days.

Soothing moisture for inflamed skin and rashes

    1 ounce of almond milk
    Essential oils:
    2 drops of lavender
    1 drop of blue chamomile

Mix essential oils into a glass container, then pour in almond milk and stir. Blue chamomile will not mix completely in milk, so you must agitate vigorously. Smooth over clean or steamed skin with circular, upward strokes. Let dry; do not rinse.

Healing milk for oily skin with acne

    1 ounce of almond milk
    Essential oils:
    4 drops of lemon
    2 drop of clary sage
    1 drop of lavender
    1 drop of rose otto

Mix essential oils in a glass container. Stir in milk, shaking vigorously. Smooth over steamed skin with circular, upward, gentle strokes. Let dry; do not rinse.

Frequently, oily skin and skins with acne are brutally treated with harsh chemicals and intense scrubbing. Acne often happens in very emotionally sensitive people, for whom the practice of self-acceptance and love is an issue. Rose otto is a luxury, soothing the emotions, and at the same time it is a mild astringent helping to correct excessive oil on the skin.

The Masks

These are the most vital, perishable, and luxurious skin applications. Use organically grown ingredients if possible and avoid mixing in containers made of aluminum or wood. Wait for your pamper day to mix these, when you can take time out and treat your skin to a super nourishment while you relax. These nourishing masks are at their best on the day they are mixed; however, they will still be effective for one or two more days if refrigerated. Use mask by itself, or as part of a facial. You can use the leftover on your body after exfoliating with a fiber brush.

Emerald Moss

Anti-inflammatory, aromatic, live green gel to nourish inflamed/acne skins. Oily and normal skins may use this formula as a firming gel.

> 1 T of tomato pulp
> ¼ cup of boiling water
> 1 T of comfrey root powder
> 10 almonds
> 1 t of spirulina
> 1 t of slippery elm powder
> *Essential oils:*
> 3 drops of lemon
> 2 drops of tea tree
> 2 drops of rosemary verbanon
> 1 drop of blue chamomile
> 1 drop of peppermint

How to do it:

1. Soak comfrey root in the ¼ cup of boiling water while you prepare the almond milk by the quick method: pour more boiling water on almonds and let it sit until water is lukewarm; drain water out and push almonds out of skins and place all 10 peeled almonds in the blender to wait while you prepare all other ingredients.
2. Strain tomato pulp into a bowl, separating seeds and skin.
3. Measure 1 T of tomato pulp and place it in a bowl.
4. Mix spirulina into the tomato pulp with a small spoon until smooth, then add the slippery elm continuously mixing until smooth.
5. Add essential oils and keep stirring.
6. Stir comfrey root water, then drain through a strainer, adding this mucilaginous water to the almonds in the blender; blend at high speed until homogeneous.
7. Strain to collect ¼ cup of liquid. You can add a little water to the pulp to complete this measurement if needed.
8. Add this almond/comfrey liquid very slowly, continuously stirring, to the rest of recipe until homogeneous. You should end up with a smooth, translucent, green gel; let it sit for a minute before applying on dry skin. Let mask dry completely before removing with a steaming hot, wrung-out washcloth, using gentle upward circular strokes. Rinse face in cool water and air dry.

Papaya / Almond Sea Foam

Luxurious nourishing mask for dry and sensitive skins.

10 presoaked almonds
1 T of papaya pulp
1 t of dulse flakes
½ cup of rejuvelac
½ t of slippery elm
½ t of honey
1 capsule of vitamin E
Essential Oils:
6 drops of sandalwood
2 drops of neroli
1 drop of Roman chamomile
1 drop of blue chamomile

How to do it:

1. Rinse dulse flakes in warm water and place with the almonds into the rejuvelac.
2. Blend for two minutes at high speed, strain and let sit while you prepare the other ingredients.
3. Mix papaya pulp, slippery elm, honey and vitamin E.
4. Mix essential oils into liquid from step 2, then pour it into the rest of mixture, stirring until smooth. Apply mask to dry skin and let it dry completely before wiping off with a steaming hot, wrung-out wash cloth with gentle, circular, upward strokes; rinse with lukewarm water, ending with a final cool splash or floral spray.

Strawberry Rose Glow

Nourishing/calming mask for normal skin.

  1 T of strawberry pulp
  1 T of barley flour
  ½ t of fresh almond milk
  ½ t of rejuvelac (see recipes on page 113)
  ½ t of honey
  Essential oils:
  2 drops of rose otto
  1 drop of lavender
  1 drop of neroli

How to do it:

1. Mix strawberry pulp with barley flour.
2. Mix almond milk with rejuvelac.
3. Mix honey with essential oils.
4. Mix step 1, 2, and 3 and stir until smooth. Apply on dry face and let it dry completely; wipe off with a steaming hot, wrung-out washcloth with gentle, circular, upward strokes; rinse with lukewarm water, with a final cool splash or spray.

The Hot Oil Hair Treatment

This treatment opens the hair follicles, giving the essential oils a chance to work deep down to the roots, stimulating circulation. Leaves hair pliable and shiny. Use once a month to maintain healthy hair and keep split ends from proliferating.

Normal, dry and damaged hair (makes one application):

> 1 T of jojoba oil
> ½ T of avocado oil
> ½ T of aloe vera oil
> *Essential oils:*
> 10 drops of rosemary
> 6 drops of lavender
> 3 drops of geranium
> 1 drop of peppermint

First mix vegetable oils in a double boiler or a fondue/crock pot and heat to about 70° F. Remove from heat and add essential oils, stirring to mix. For long hair, dip ends of brushed hair into hot oil and carefully spread oil to rest of hair, massaging upward towards scalp. Put hair into a plastic cap and cover with a warm towel. Leave for at least 30 minutes, brushing again with a comb and shampooing twice to remove all oil. For short hair, apply oil as hot as your hands can stand to hair, and follow the same procedure.

Infant Massage Oil

To make one ounce:

> ¼ oz of aloe vera oil
> ½ oz of rice bran oil
> ¼ oz of hazelnut oil
> *Essential Oils:*
> 3 drops of blue chamomile
> 7 drops of lavender.

Shake it all together.

For more recipes and education on homemade cosmetics, see Appendix.

MEDICAL AROMATHERAPY

Therapies using essential oils are not to be understood with the same attitude of "instant results" in the way they are expected from allopathic medicine. However, in my own life, I have noticed amazingly fast results at certain times.

In medical aromatherapy, essential oils are ingested, used as suppositories, inhaled, or applied on the skin—on the whole body or localized areas—through massage. The aromatic molecules penetrate the body, entering the blood stream via the skin by massage, via the lungs by inhalation, and via the digestive system by ingestion or suppository application.

Certain oils can cross the blood-brain barrier, reach the brain tissue, and cause damage to nerve and tissue. These toxic oils can be used therapeutically; that is the reason why education in medical aromatherapy is crucial before it is used as a system for self-treatment.

Doctors such as Dr. Jean Valnet, Dr. Jean Claude Lapraz, Dr. Daniel Pénoël, and research scientist Pierre Franchomme, who are expert in the medical use of essential oils, tour from Europe to the United States and teach medical aromatherapy. In France, aromatherapy is a course offered in pharmaceutical and medical schools.

One of the most important things that happens when one uses aromatherapy, is that it puts the individual in touch with a form of holistic healing that addresses more than the physical body in a very tangible way, through smell. For example: lemon oil is a strong antiseptic that can protect the body's respiratory system from infection. As the lemon oil is addressing the respiratory infection, at the same time its sedative properties have an effect on the nervous system. So, by affecting the emotions to calm the individual, the mind will settle and be directed to another experience, through the olfactory system. The aroma of the lemon oil will distract the mind from discomfort and let the body do the healing.

This constitutes a pleasurable way to deal with illness, which in the long run pays off on many levels. Currently a few physicians are using aromatherapy in their practices.

Some oils can be applied without dilution. Among those, lavender and tea tree are some of the most important oils because of their wide range of properties. Some oils are safe to apply neat (without dilution) to certain tissue but not another tissue. Even oils that are non-toxic can aggravate and cause discomfort to certain tissue. For example, one can use rosemary oil inside the nostrils as a decongestant, but it will be inappropriate to use it neat on the armpits, as it could cause a burning sensation.

Citrus oils, including bergamot, should never be used in preparations involving sun exposure, as they are photosensitive and can permanently stain the skin.

Preparations for babies and pregnant women need different considerations, as well.

A good habit to develop to test for sensitivity is to always apply a blend on a small area of the skin before applying oils, even diluted, on a larger area of the body.

Hypotensive individuals should avoid the oils that activate blood circulation, such as basil, peppermint, or rosemary.

There is so much to know on the medical uses of essential oils that a book such as this one cannot possibly cover all the necessary facts. Please refer to the Appendix for more books on the subject and sources for continuing education.

MEDICINAL TRAVEL KIT

Following is a small and safe essential oil kit I use for simple therapies while I am traveling. I acquired this medical aromatherapy knowledge by studying with Pierre Franchomme and Dr. Pénoël, and experimenting for a number of years.

Essential oils in the kit, 5 milliliters each:

basil, bergamot, blue chamomile, clary sage, eucalyptus, frankincense, geranium, lavender, lemon, neroli, peppermint, Roman chamomile, *Rosa damascena*, rosemary, sandalwood, tea tree, ylang ylang.

Abdominal pain and intestinal gas: use 6 drops of peppermint oil, variety *Mentha piperita* only, in ½ ounce of vegetable oil. Massage the area every two hours and drink peppermint tea. Four drops of *Mentha piperita* oil can be ingested or used as a suppository, inside gelatin capsules (never in teas), 2 times each day.

Aching muscles: Massage oil of 15 drops of lavender oil and two drops of blue chamomile oil in 1 ounce of vegetable oil.

Athlete's foot: Dab tea tree oil, neat, onto the foot, every hour.

Burns, cuts, insect bites: Dab lavender oil, neat, on the affected area.

Bladder irritations: These therapies will provide relief and comfort for bladder infections and keep them from getting worse. If allopathic drugs such as antibiotics are used, these essential oil therapies can be used at the same time. It is very good and strengthening to keep these oils flowing through the bladder and stay connected with your plant oil allies. Drink 2 to 3 quarts per day of bladder irritation tea (page 138). Multiply the recipe to make a gallon for a sitz bath before bedtime.

Boils and skin infections: Support tissue with applications of lavender or tea tree oil. Both can be applied, undiluted, directly on inflamed tissue. This will keep the area clean, and keep infections from spreading further, supporting the formation of scar tissue. If skin is very inflamed and fairly red, add one drop of blue chamomile oil to the lavender or tea tree. If you insist, it won't persist.

Congested sinuses and respiratory infections: For inhalation, apply 1 drop eucalyptus oil, 2 drops rosemary oil, and 5 drops lemon oil to steaming hot water and inhale as much as possible under a towel, with closed eyes. Repeat this treatment every 4 hours. It is also nice to mix two parts lemon oil with one part eucalyptus oil and use a couple of drops on a cloth to inhale during the course of the day. Drink colds, flus and respiratory infections tea (page 138).

Food poisoning: Mix 4 drops of lemon oil into a teaspoon of honey and pour hot water over it to make tea. One can drink up to three cups a day. This tea can also be used as a preventive to protect one from contracting contagious infections, such as in seasonal flu epidemics.

Herpes simplex: Mix one part eucalyptus oil with one part tea tree oil and apply neat with fingertip on sore every hour, with vitamin E oil in between, to support the tissue while the sore is being dried up by constant application of the oils. It dulls the edge of pain and heals in one week instead of two. If you have rose otto and geranium oils, these are an even more efficient therapy for herpes simplex. Follow the same instructions; just substitute the oils. This second combination is much milder on the lip tissue. It may even have a faster healing time, and the vitamin E can be nice, but it is not as necessary.

Headaches: Apply lavender oil with a drop of peppermint oil on temples, on the back of the neck and between the nose and the upper lip. At night, put two drops of lavender oil on the pillow. Drink insomnia tea (page 138) or precious flower tea (page 139).

Insomnia: Apply a couple drops of lavender to your pillow.

Mental fatigue: Make a hot footbath with 6 drops of rosemary oil. Rub a couple of undiluted drops of peppermint oil between the palms of your hands, cup your hands over your nose and inhale deeply. Avoid getting peppermint oil in your eyes. Peppermint will not damage your eyes, but it will deliver a strong burning sensation for quite some time.

Nausea and motion sickness: Use lavender, basil, or peppermint oil for inhalation by pouring a couple of drops in a handkerchief to sniff during bouts of motion sickness or other types of nausea. You can use a drop or two of these same oils in an Aromajewel, if you have one, to inhale while traveling.

PMS and uterine cramps: Mix 1 drop of blue chamomile oil and 2 drops of lavender oil with 5 drops of clary sage oil into ½ ounce of vegetable oil. Massage the mixture on the lower abdomen. Avoid this treatment during pregnancy. Drink precious flower tea (page 139).

Sunburn: Mix 10 drops of lavender in ½ ounce of aloe vera oil or almond oil and apply gently.

Vaginal dryness: Mix two parts jojoba or coconut oil and one part melted cocoa butter to make 1 ounce. Add to this mixture 3 drops of sandalwood oil and 1 drop rose otto or neroli oil. Stir while warm to an even mix. Allow it to cool to solidify. Smooth the balm with fingers on skin, two times a day and before intercourse. Completely safe. Yum.

Making Tea with Essential Oils

I have developed a habit of making tea using essential oils.

Although it may be an acquired taste for some, and involve a previous dilution of the essential oil into a tablespoon of vodka, brandy, or other alcohol prior to mixing with hot water, tea turns out to be a great way to use oils for simple therapies while traveling.

In my suggested kit, essential oils that are good for tea preparation are basil, bergamot, Roman chamomile, lavender, lemon, neroli, rose and tea tree.

While traveling, I find it advantageous to use essential oils instead of herbs, because essential oils do not have a shelf life like herbs do, and occupy a lot less space. I have always found it valuable to have a few 5ml bottles of oil while traveling. (Avoid using styrofoam cups, because essential oils will carve holes in the cup; choose glass or porcelain.) This practice has always made my trip more pleasant and energized. I have found it to be a great help to have the life-giving qualities of plant oils close at hand, as my allies, during my travels. Oftentimes, people sitting next to me also enjoyed the aroma, and I would end up answering questions and giving a mini-lecture on essential oils to the curious neighbors...

Essential oils in the correct measure can be mixed into sugar and alcohol and dispersed in hot water to create a pleasant drink. However, the essential oils will not completely dissipate into the water, so expect to see oil floating on surface of your tea—some more than others, depending on the volatility of each oil—but if the recipe is done carefully, this should not be a problem. The more volatile oils, such as lavender, peppermint or rose, have a fine dispersion. The citrus oils lemon and bergamot require stirring prior to drinking each time. Good teas to drink while traveling are basil, Roman chamomile, lavender, lemon, neroli, peppermint, rose otto and tea tree. My favorite tea for supporting my digestive system is a combination of Roman chamomile oil with basil oil, or just plain basil. To sleep, lavender with Roman chamomile or rose otto is an effective tea.

Preparing Essential Oil Teas

Mix the desired oil into one or two teaspoons of sugar, mixing vigorously to distribute evenly. Slowly add one tablespoon of vodka and then one cup of hot water, pouring hot water over sugar slowly, continuously mixing. Oils will not disperse completely in the water, but the dispersion after careful mixing is good enough to drink pleasantly. Citrus oils may require to be stirred again prior to drinking. One can use honey or maple syrup instead of sugar, but it will be a little more difficult to do the mixing.

Essential Oil Tea Recipes

These recipes have been tested, using completely safe oils for digestion.

Bladder irritation

3 drops bergamot
6 drops tea tree

Colds, flus and respiratory infections

2 drops lemon
6 drops tea tree

Diarrhea

2 drops basil
1 drop Roman chamomile

Flatulence

1 drop peppermint

Insomnia

1 drop lavender
½ drop Roman chamomile
or use a simple
lavender tea with 2 drops of lavender

Nausea and motion sickness

1 drop peppermint
2 drops basil

PMS, anxiety, nervous tension

Use precious flower tea or rose otto tea.

Precious flower tea

2 drops lavender
1 drop rose otto
1 drop neroli (optional)
2 t sugar
1 T vodka, brandy or wine
4 cups hot water

Rose otto tea

1 drop rose otto
2 cups water
2 t sugar
1 T vodka, brandy or wine

The two teas above are sedatives, and they work great hot or chilled. Essential oil teas, especially the precious flower ones, mature lovely in the refrigerator overnight. Try them chilled on a hot afternoon, with ice and a sprig of peppermint. Voila! A fantastic wine substitute. Therapeutic properties remain, and they will create very exotic party drinks.

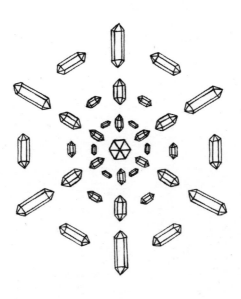

Merkabah Crystal Grid

PART TWO

Crystals

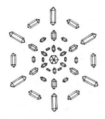

...as were they indeed living things, they rejoiced in light and received it and gave it back in hues more marvelous than before.
~J.R.R. Tolkien

PHYSICAL ASPECTS OF QUARTZ CRYSTALS

Quartz crystal is a solid that precipitates from a silica-rich hydrothermal solution containing water, gases, and elements in suspension such as iron, silica, etc. This environment in the deep layers of the earth is one of high pressure and heat, and the quartz crystal initiates its growth when conditions are perfect for the bonding of the atoms. From a particular given point, let's say a start-up seed, a chain reaction occurs in the proportion of one atom of silica to two atoms of oxygen, and it begins to accumulate, multiplying and forming a molecular grid as a stack of tetrahedrons in the shape of a spiral; this construction results in a mineral with an external hexagonal form. The typical quartz crystal presents externally six sides or faces, and equal angles of 120 degrees, with three imaginary axes in different lengths, known as A, B, and C axis. This is how we can define its form. Quartz hardness is seven; harder than your teeth, which have the hardness of five.

The quartz crystal's principal property is piezoelectricity, which means "pressure electricity." Piezoelectricity is the emission of electrons from its atomic layers, in response to a stimulus, which can be mechanical or electric. When an electrical current is applied to the crystal it develops an alternating negative and positive charge, causing an oscillation that is constant. If a mechanical stimulus is applied, the quartz crystal emits a similar electrical charge. These charges can be captured with sensitive equipment. This process was discovered in 1880 by Pierre and Jacques Curie. Now we use it in all communications technologies. For example, a slice of quartz is added to certain equipment; let's say a TV tower. To this slice of quartz is applied an electrical stimulus. The quartz will produce a constant oscillation that the tower uses to emit its signals. It is the well-known "crystal oscillator" used in radio, computers, and satellites. Remember the common quartz watch, with a battery that stimulates the quartz electrically. This produces a constant mechanical oscillation that is used to measure time.

The frequency of the wave is determined by the thickness of the quartz slice. Scientifically, quartz is used to convert, stabilize, transduce, focus, record, transfer, regulate, or modulate. The most interesting thing to me is that in our modern technology quartz is used to help us in *communications*; the dissemination of organized energies from one location to another, utilizing and producing light, electricity, sound, ultrasound, or information. This technology translates to many fields of action, such as medicine and ultrasonic submarine detectors, as well as metaphysical light technologies. We will explore the metaphysical aspects later.

Refraction, Attenuation and Color in Natural Stones: How the Crystal Creates Rainbows. Why is a Ruby Red?

Naturally colored stones, as well as colorless stones such as quartz and diamond, are physical forms containing the highest rate of vibrations from the mineral kingdom. Colorless stones like quartz and diamond transmit all the frequency rates of the spectrum, all colors, so they are light itself; frozen light. These colorless stones can create a prismatic effect. The prismatic effect depends on the property of attenuation and refraction to produce rainbows. Attenuation, the opposite of amplification, occurs when light encounters very dense matter such as a crystal. The light that is speeding through the atmosphere slows down and bends at an angle as it penetrates the crystal's atomic structure. This bending of the light creates the separation of the colors of the spectrum, and that is the prismatic rainbow that we see. All the colors each have different rates of vibration and different speeds, or rather, wave lengths. That is how the colors separate. Colors vibrate at different rates as the light penetrates the crystal. Refraction is the angle of bending of the light, which is different for each color. The colors fan out, creating a rainbow. Lower frequencies are the reds and oranges moving up to the yellows, and higher frequencies are the greens, blues, indigos.

In many ways, light can be understood as communicating information.

An ordinary way to exemplify this is with a dark room: we have no idea of the colors or shapes of objects in it. As soon as we turn on the light we see it all almost instantaneously. When we focus on a stone, it provides us with vast amounts of information on numerous levels of our perception, conscious and unconscious. This process is extremely individual, because each person operates at a different level of sensitivity.

Trace-metal elements in the crystal structure, plus their interaction with light, are what make the color of a stone. Let's learn about spectro-transmission and spectro-absorption. Full spectro-transmission means that the light is being transmitted through the stone. Full spectro-absorption means that the stone is absorbing all the light that is moving through the stone. These are the black stones, such as black jade or black tourmaline. The color of a stone depends on at what vibratory rate a stone absorbs the light.

For example: Ruby is red; that means the only part of the spectrum transmitted out of the stone is the red ray. The stone is absorbing all the other rays of the spectrum, the greens and the blues, etc. So, a stone is really serving the specialized purpose of transmitting that particular ray of the light that is also in alliance with the chemical composition and trace metals of the stone, to the surrounding environment.

The light goes in and vibrates in the stone. The stone is at a certain frequency due to its chemical composition and structure. The light that comes out is the reflection of the frequency of the light that is being transmitted. If the red part of the spectrum which is a slower vibration than the greens, blues and violets, is what is being held in the stone, then what is going to be transmitted is a color at a higher frequency than red, which could be a green or another higher-frequency color. A blue stone, such as an aquamarine, is an example. This is only mentioning the colors that are perceived by the naked eye, without going into the ultraviolets or infrareds, which our vision does not perceive.

A Metaphysical Perspective on Quartz Crystals

Some of us have a vision of the universe as an interconnected network of interdimensional crystalline code patterns. When worlds are not physical they exist as blueprints, holding possibilities as the consciousness of the universe travels through worlds, manifesting in different frequency or layers. "Crystalline" is a way to define a organized field of energy that can communicate between dimensions and transduce, replicate, convert, stabilize, focus, record, transfer, regulate, modulate; all the abilities of the quartz crystal that we talked about previously.

I began to be interested in these matters at the same time that I became an avid student and researcher of aromatherapy and plant-source essential oils. At that time, at the beginning of the '80s, I also developed a great interest in the work of Randall and Vicki Baer (*The Crystal Connection; A Guide Book to Personal and Planetary Ascension,* and *Windows of Light; Quartz Crystals and Self-Transformation*). I had already been working with quartz crystals and minerals, together with my husband Brian Cook. Brian was purveying world-class minerals to museums and we were living with an energetic form of life that was affecting us a great deal. Brian also was importing quartz crystals from the mines of Minas Gerais, Bahia and Goias, the extraordinary rich Brazilian soil. We would receive shipments of quartz crystals in barrels and have impromptu "crystal gazing" nights. The crystals would arrive all wrapped up in newspapers. We would each grab one to unwrap, ready for each surprising character to reveal their fabulous crystallizations: beautiful points, hexagonal crystal bodies with symmetrical and asymmetrical features, long, short, skinny, fat, double-terminated, mother crystals with babies growing on them, amazing phantom inclusions, etc... We would notice crystallization depicting lines and patterns that would make me feel like a certain divine intelligence was communicating with us with petrified records.

At that time I was also studying mineralogy and crystallography with Brian from a more scientific perspective, and I wanted to create a bridge between the scientific and the metaphysical views. I wanted to take scientific facts and see them in another light. What I was gathering from studying crystallography was that the greatest underlining principle had all to do with numbers, angles, and geometry. Randall would talk about codes of light and blueprints, and how there is a dimensionally-interconnecting crystalline pattern that runs through the entire universe. My own insight was telling me to create specific harmonics by arranging crystals in grids that obeyed the numeric relationship found in each particular mineral system. The idea was that the grids are signaling stations that could communicate interdimensionally.

The center of a grid, according to Randall and Vicky, has the capacity to generate a magnetic field that dimensionally would be perceived as a pillar of light. To set up a grid one has to construct a geometric arrangement, positioning stones in a symmetric pattern, sometimes with a center. This organizes the crystals, creating a unified field of energy.

I was thinking of possibilities going back to the Stone Age people. Science would attempt to understand Stone Age people as working to create calendars and clocks by the placement of megalithic stones in relationship with the sun, moon and visible stars; but I was considering even more the fact that a mechanism could be set up for interdimensional communications. The physical world, being the densest matter, can be seen as a very useful point of reference interdimensionally, a place for convergence of different types of energy. Made sense to me that we would use quartz crystals—solid objects that have configurations for working with light. This view was like meditating on the vast possibilities of the consciousness of the universe.

From the scientific world I was getting important facts: Every mineral as it forms obeys its own angles, number of faces and form. There are seven crystal systems: **triclinic**, **monoclinic**, **hexagonal**, **orthorhombic**, **rhombohedral**, **tetragonal** and **isometric**.

As my fascination grew, I began to select certain mineral shapes fit for the construction of grids. However, since it was very difficult to find the stones, I invested in precision faceting equipment that could cut these particular mineral shapes using very clear optical quartz.

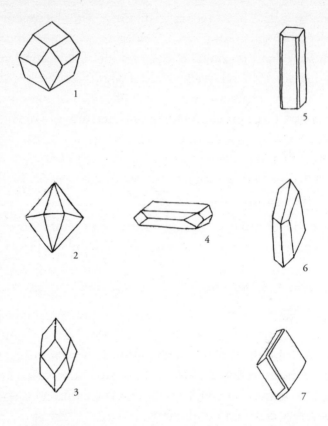

The Seven Crystals Systems—Geometry of Nature!

1. Isometric System represented by a Garnet
2. Hexagonal System represented by a Beta Quartz
3. Tetragonal System represented by an Apophyllite
4. Orthohombic System represented by an a Barite
5. Triclinic System represented by an a Kyanite
6. Monoclinic System represented by an a Selenite
7. Rhombohedral System represented by an a Rhodochrosite

For studies on the angles, refer to *Manual of Mineralogy* by Cornelius Hurlbut and Cornelis Klein.

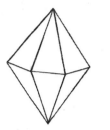
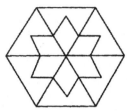

External View   *Internal View*

STARGEMS

At that time, I was living in between the USA and Brazil, and it was the end of the '80s. I became very aware of a certain crystal form that looks like two quartz points stuck together without a body, a bi-pyramidal form (see Figure above). I could see this shape everywhere in artwork, cartoons, etc... and looking for it in the gem & mineral shows, I could never find it. Brian explained to me that that shape corresponded to the "beta" quartz, a high-temperature form of quartz that only occurs around volcanoes. I chose this shape to concentrate on for my grids. I learned how to make paper models with Mr. Tesandro, a professor of crystallography at the Federal University of Bahia. With the paper model, we created a numeric formula to be able to program my precision cutting machine. To my intense surprise, when the first crystal was cut, and I was examining it, I notice that if one looked from one point to the other, one could see a hexagonal star forming in the center of the crystal, the geometry of the familiar Star of David.

It reminded me of the "golden mean," which defines the harmonic aspect found in nature that repeats itself with a geometric proportion, such as the nautilus shell, snowflakes, sunflowers, etc… The consciousness of the universe thinks in mathematical codes, perhaps to be able to record, amplify and transmit energy, and manipulate matter. (For more information on the golden mean, read a wonderful book called *The Power of Limits* by Gyorgy Doczi.) Nature created a geometry that depicted, inside a quartz crystal, a hexagonal star! The very star that has been recognized by Judaism, Hinduism and Buddhism, that symbolizes the perfect harmonious aspect of the union of energy and matter, and the polarities of positive and negative, Yin and Yang. For many years these crystals became my obsession. I called them "Stargems."

It was intriguing to me to notice the myriads of geometric forms that minerals take on the earth. My view of life became permeated with geometry, proportions, and harmonics; everywhere I looked and everything I did and talked about was geometry and the consciousness of the universe. The message was in everything! The design of city buildings, park plans, landscape of gardens, credit cards' size; everything around us was connected to this intrinsic knowledge. To me it was an obvious language from nature, just like the scent from the plant essential oils was a language from nature.

I had a late friend who was a Cherokee Indian shaman in his seventies. We called him "Grandpa Roberts." He collected stones and had a special relationship with crystals. He was not a scientist, but always transmitted the feeling of being certain of his knowledge. He influenced my knowing how to live with crystals and stones without the never-ending desire to understand, explain, and define. His way was one of perceiving, feeling and merging. Part of what drew me to him was to experience the two worlds and make a connection. I found myself getting in touch with a different way to understand communication with nature, a different way to see. This way did not need the logical mind to process, to achieve an intellectual satisfaction. The understanding of an observation can be done in a scientific way, by using the logical mind to understand, like a "spotlight," an ordinary, sharp vision. There is another way, a "diffuse light," a gestalt vision, that is more like awareness, like a diffuse floodlight. I learned that both ways can be a true view of reality, and we are free to choose.

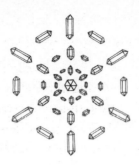

GRIDWORKS

My deepest interest in the metaphysical perspective remained with the work of Randall and Vicki, which delivered information about a future light technology aimed towards personal and planetary ascension. Their work was, in turn, greatly influenced by J.J. Hurtak (*The Book of Knowledge; The Keys of Enoch*). Randall and Vicki were teaching about gridworks, and their information interfaced like a glove with my own personal inner discoveries and spontaneously rising understanding.

Quartz crystals were the mineral that we were all working with. It comes with a clear crystalline structure; it can deflect light into rainbows, and has a spiral chemical structure that corresponds with our DNA. Those were exciting times. Randall and Vicki would talk about bringing information for a type of future technology. They were teaching us how to set up a "Merkabah" grid, placing 36 double-terminated quartz crystals of different sizes into a hexagonal mandala. It was another, more complex, Star of David! This was the grid that mostly interested me, because it coincided with my idea of arranging the crystals in a configuration obeying that particular mineral system. It was hexagonal and had the hexagonal quartz crystals forming it. This crystal mandala geometry was extraordinary.

I was living in Brazil for a couple of years and we were buying stones, collecting, and visiting mines all over. I wanted to find a large number of double-terminated crystals that were clear, undamaged and in all the sizes to compose the mandala. Believe it or not, Brian ran into someone traveling though one of the mines he was visiting, who had a large bag of all the double-terminated crystals that had just been mined in another area. Brian brought them all to me. The bag contained three times or more the number of crystals I was looking for. It took me a good number of days to classify them all by clarity and size. One day I finally had the perfect 36 crystals for the grid. Now I could begin to put the symmetric hexagonal grid together (see the diagram at the beginning of this part).

This first effort took many, many hours. I started after lunch and when the sun went down and it was night, I was finished. The crystals were sitting on a piece of hard cardboard covered with a sky-blue silk cloth. As I got the numbers, sizes and line configurations together, I became very sensitive to the effect of the alignment of the crystal lines. It was like I had put together some type of mechanism. I could feel the harmonics of a certain resonance that had a perceptible vibration. Looking back to the remaining crystals from the original bag, all unwrapped and lying on the floor in disarray, I could easily feel the difference between that and what I had put together. The crystals in disarray didn't have a perceptible harmonic resonance.

After I finished this Merkabah crystal grid setup, I was exhausted and easily felt asleep on my bed, right by the grid's side. Began to dream a brilliant, conscious dream. I am arriving at a place like Stonehenge, except that the stones are all clear crystals. As I approach the crystals closer I notice that they are lying in a circular form. I realize that I am walking in between the crystals of a giant Merkabah grid, just like the one I had just finished setting up. I enter the grid and begin to walk between the crystals, towards the center of the grid. As I approach the center, I feel a tremendous centrifugal force pulling me into a tunnel of light. I wake up with a start! Uf! Amazing and very intense!

Now I can set up the Merkabah grid in 15 minutes, and have been doing it in different places to create a harmonic resonance and send an interdimensional signal throughout the universe, linking our earth with other layers of consciousness.

In a very human, practical way, creating harmonics with a powerful resonance of a crystal grid is the most superior tool for meditation and healing. The human body is positively affected by harmonic resonance. It has the tendency to align the different layers of energy in the human body; the physical, emotional, mental and spiritual levels, all working to create a complete whole. When unbalances and staggered energies occur, we have disharmony and disease. A harmonic resonance is a powerful restructuring influence.

A Story of Healing Using a Crystal

I was traveling in Hawaii and ran across a woman in great pain and suffering from a past miscarriage. She felt very far from health. She had hemorrhage and infection, and a lot of fear and anxiety around when it would all be over, and if she would ever be back to normal. I had a crystal that I used for programming information, so I told her to think of a reasonable time that she could believe she would be healed. We decided on a date three weeks later, and both visualized that date trapped in the lattice of the crystal. Holding the crystal with my right hand, and releasing the information from the lattice with a strong exhalation and intent, we both visualized the information transferring to her DNA from the crystal lattice. At the end of the third week, I received a letter from her saying "Here I am at the post office sending you this note. This is the precise date and I am on my feet!"

Oftentimes people have an idea that the crystal itself has powers, almost as if we can set a crystal down and it will do some miraculous thing. Nothing could be further from the truth, for the power of a crystal to serve as a tool depends on our interaction and synergy, with what is in our minds and the crystalline structure combined. One does not depend on faith, but if there is mistrust, that feeling can cancel out possibilities of healing.

In primitive times, someone had to have the idea that the milk from goats could feed humans also, and that a donkey could transport goat milk from one settlement to another. It all begins with an internal impulse to think, experiment, and create a situation using a tool; whole systems can be created after that.

LIQUID CRYSTALS

IBM scientist Marcel Vogel, Ph.D., of the Psychic Research Institute in San Jose, California, researched liquid crystals extensively. He was able to measure in his lab, through various spectrographic analyses, that we can create change in matter with our thoughts. Our thoughts create a measurable vibration that can have an influence on matter such as water, stones, our bodies, or other biological systems. Marcel used crystals as a means to transfer thoughts to water, and was also able to measure changes in aluminum conductivity, surface tension, ultraviolet frequencies, etc.

Liquid crystals, which we have in our bodies, are a state between a solid and a liquid. A liquid crystal is equal to a quartz crystal, in that it is a highly-organized chemical structure that can reproduce itself and transfer information between molecules via photonic emission, light, or electromagnetic radiation. Liquid crystals communicate information between our cells within our biological systems. Quartz crystal can receive vibratory information from thoughts into its geometric chemical lattice structure and communicate it to another unified field of energy. The concept is like a computer function where you have an image, the icon representing the stored information, which you can drag with the mouse to another application. Information can be transferred efficiently, without loss of energy.

How to Care for, Clean, Charge, and Activate Crystals

How to care for a crystal

Quartz crystals have the ability to store and hold information, so it is important to delete all previous charges from time to time to get rid of the accumulation. Have a clear focus and great awareness of intention when handling them. Choose to place crystals in an undisturbed area where they are safe from bumping on things and chipping. The chipping of their bodies can diminish their capacity. If you have so many crystals that it becomes difficult to care properly for all of them, choose one or a few at a time, so you can always have each one at its maximum capacity.

How to clean and clear

One of the best ways to clean crystals is to bury them in salt, or place them into a very strong solution of salt and water, and rinse under running water.

I like to use a powerful forced exhale with a strong intention of clearing a crystal (Marcel Vogel's technique) to delete all psychic energies that may be contained in it, and another exhale to program a given intention.

Try to clean your crystals every week or every waxing moon.

Charging and activating

To charge a crystal means to start over with a maximum capacity for storage of vibrational information: thoughts, feelings, visualized images. A great way to charge a crystal is to place it the center of a grid or inside a pyramid. One can also use a laser light for at least 10 minutes, or place crystals outdoors in a power spot or sacred place.

To activate and expand the crystal's capabilities of interfacing with the universal crystalline grid, place the crystal in the elemental influences of nature: in rainfall, storms, lightning; by the sea, springs and streams; under full moons. The natural resonance of quartz interfaces with the resonance of the earth. There is a natural record of the earth's resonance in the crystal, similar to the way we carry genetic codes from our parents in our DNA. Therefore, it is a wonderful way to clear, charge and activate a crystal all at once, by burying the crystal in the earth for a period of time from a couple of days to a moon phase, or whatever comes to you intuitively at the time.

Aromajewels

Crystals and natural-colored stones or gems are the highest frequency of the mineral kingdom. Likewise, essential oils are the distilled elixir of the highest vibration from the plant kingdom; the volatile, the spirit of the plant. When we humans synergize these two powers together and apply it to our energy fields, it creates a strong influence from the highest earth frequency in our electromagnetic circuitry. It is impossible not to be affected with all kinds of magnetic information and light emissions. But why do we do these things? I think we are living an era when we are very active in our will to become aware of much more than we have been, in ourselves and with the environment. These new experiences are here to create more possibilities for us, and it all has to do with perceiving invisible vibrational realities, which we begin to know when we became more aware and sensitive to ourselves and our environment.

At this point I feel like sharing with you my experience of creating my line of aromatic stones and jewelry called Aromajewels.®

My first thought about creating Aromajewels held an ancient feeling...almost as if I was hearing whispers of the past coming from the future. It had that timeless quality and experience of harmonious wonder that I often feel when I am

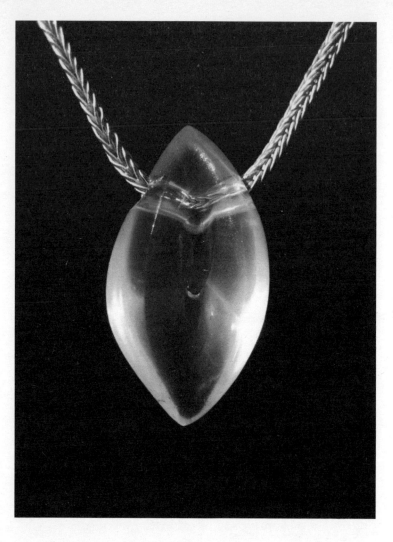

Rose Quartz Aromajewel Flame Pendant with Rose Otto

working with stones and with essential oils, but putting the two together in a synergy really lifted me to a exalted state of consciousness, something like riding on a forever-flying magic carpet. It is really difficult to explain this feeling. Words easily fail to describe the enormous pleasure of experiencing such stones on my body and energy field.

All the time I would spend with my first Aromajewels, I could feel nature working with me in the elementals of plant and mineral, and became accustomed to receiving information from their fields. In reciprocity, I felt that the human element of thought and intention, manifested as the design and manufacture, which I provided to make this entity a physical reality, was a source of joy in the other dimensions involved also. Together we perceived the workings of a fabulous synergy! The Aromajewel was better than the essential oil in the bottle was better than the rough piece of stone and it was better than my thoughts, drawings and wax models. Together we did it! We created a synergy of the best natural elements from the mineral and plant kingdoms as a gift to the human world.

Shortly after inventing Aromajewels, I went to homes and shows bringing an exciting treasure box filled with these fragrant gems. I would do "show and tell" events. People were delighted, marveling at the new invention and expressing a certain inner recognition for these amulet-type jewels, almost as if they had created them themselves. They recognized them; something in them was so familiar, the seduction of a certain magic, something that spoke with the language of spirit. People were inspired to relax, hold a stone, breathe natural fragrance, and share this experience with someone special to them.

Why did a simple piece of jewelry create such heated interest? One could think: smell. Fragrance coming from the heart of a gem.

In smelling, one has to focus. By focusing with smell, the mind stops its never-ending thoughts. This is an anti-stress activity, just like sitting in a beautiful garden. This garden visit can happen in the middle of congested traffic in the city, with true aromas from nature, essential oils, coming from the jewel. It is like a security blanket that connects us to our basic support system, nature. The value in connecting to nature is for the self-empowerment of merging with something greater than ourselves, Earth, the divinity that we can touch physically. Gems and crystals are a concentrated and specialized earth, with a precious message.

Aromajewels have the power to unite the value of precious earth elements, gems and fragrance from nature, and transmit that synergy to our energy fields. Plants have intelligence. They exhale oxygen, and give us life. Pure smells that are true from nature can be safely inhaled over and over again, contrary to synthetic perfume smells that can go against our well-being. Aromatic plants have a special power among all plants; they have a specific language from Mother Nature when she is teaching us about healing and feeling good.

Earth Diving Meditation

I suggest that you make a recording of yourself reading the text below, then play it and relax as you listen:

Take your whole body, and starting from the feet, tense all your muscles; feet, legs, thighs, hips, abdomen, chest, arms, neck, face, scalp, and holding everything really tight, begin to slowly let go from the feet up, feet…legs…knees…thighs… hips…abdomen…chest…arms…neck…face…scalp… And now, with everything really soft, drop down to the feeling of gravity below you and get your consciousness to focus on your breath, feel the air going in and out of your lungs, deliciously slow and deep…the air goes in and out… Now take your consciousness to your dematerialized body, your spirit, your energy body, the life force that runs through your physical body, and focus your attention on the point of light in you…that point of light will gravitate from the point of reference that is your physical body and penetrate through the floor of this room, going further down through the grass, the wet earth with all the organic things that are living on it…and penetrate through the compressed layers of sandstone that go for miles and miles…and here you begin your journey towards the center of the earth. As you are going through the sandstone layers, you feel the dryness of these compressed layers for miles and miles, and miles…and as you go further down it begins to get quite hot, but it feels comfortable to you because you are dematerialized. Now you are reaching areas where the formation of all minerals takes place, the laboratory of the earth…you are seeing metamorphic rocks and shapes beginning to crystallize in great heat and pressure…

later to rise in an upward movement towards the surface, where they will eventually be exposed and meet erosion.

You are beginning to examine the different mineral shapes displaying their sacred geometries...and going further down you encounter a sea of molten raw lava, metals, elemental fire. At this point you are receiving an intense form of nourishment from this elemental earth in the fine channels of your energy body... Now you are perceiving golden light coming from the formation of the noble metal gold. This is a potent form of vibrational medicine that you are finding near the center of the earth... Now you get to the core. Reaching the center, you see a sphere crystallized into beautiful facets, shining like the light of a giant diamond, and it has its own light, concealed within the earth like an internal sun. It feels like a heart and a mind that has the records of the experience of all life, on and in the earth. Now it's your time to make an impression of this moment when your consciousness relates to the center of your matrix, the heart of your mother. And you tell the earth who you are now, in this very fresh moment of conscious thought, I am alive, I am awake and I am aware...and you make a connection, give the earth a special greeting. And you feel yourself become conscious and visible to this greater organism that you are a part of... And now, having made your here-and-now record of your self in the center of the earth's biological heart-mind computer-center crystal, you reverse your journey to come back, leaving the core...going through the laboratory where the minerals are in formation...and the molten lava...and the sandstone layers and finally get to the organic layer...come up to the green earth where the plants smell good and are in contact with the air, and back through the floor, and to that point of reference that is your body, and now remember your breath...air going in and out of your body...and get in touch with your muscles, begin to access your physical machine, make a wide yawn like you do in bed as you wake up in the morning.

EARTH SCIENCE INTERVIEW
WITH BRIAN COOK

This interview was done in the summer of 2006 in California, with Brian Cook, who is my husband as well as an exploration geologist and artisanal mining enthusiast. He is my walking reference on all subjects concerning the physical science of our planet. Brian is my original inspiration for studying minerals, gems and geology. He has been involved in mining projects of his own for many years, and has a deep, heartfelt sentiment for the mineral kingdom and the Earth.

The material on the profile of natural stones was derived from learning from Brian, the books in the Appendix, and my own acquired knowledge from studying and working with stones since the '70s.

Kendra:

Can you explain the different types of mining activity?

Brian:

Let us divide mining into two broad categories: Large-scale industrial mining and artisanal mining.

Large scale involves big investment companies with complex financing and institutional procedures; for example, focusing on precious-metal mines of gold, silver, platinum, palladium and diamonds, and base metals such as iron, copper, zinc, lead, tungsten, etc. The investment can be from tens of millions to billions of dollars.

The artisanal type of mining can be as basic as an individual working independently with no investment capital, to organized small companies investing from several thousands of dollars to several millions. It can include from finding any useful building materials to gold, gems and diamonds.

Kendra:

Is there a harmful environmental impact of mining, and what would that be?

Brian:

Harmful impact can be found in both corporate and artisanal levels of mining.

At the artisanal level, the harmful effect is usually related to water pollution, littering of the land, and then abandonment without reclamation.

At the corporate level the harmful effects would be the same, but on a larger scale. It is important to point out that in both types of mining, today great effort is made to address the environment through reclamation of the areas affected by the mining. This means detoxifying the water through biological creation of wetlands that scrub the toxins out of the water, at the same time adding wildlife habitats. Wealthier countries such as Canada, USA, Finland, Sweden, and most of the European countries, typically have stricter guidelines. These nations are leading the way to reclamation of the mined lands. The more profound effect of mining relates to the social impact.

Kendra:

Can you explain how mining affects our society?

Brian:

The majority of the gemstones that we see in jewelry are mined by very poor groups, all over the world, without safety precautions or regulations, in harsh environments. For the people working these mines there is usually little access to the wealth generated by the stones found. Now, in 2006, we are seeing in the gem and jewelry industry the implementation of "fair trade jewelry."

Kendra:

What is fair trade jewelry?

Brian:

Fair trade jewelry consists of people involved in the gem and jewelry industry, who are interested in re-investing in the communities where the stones are found. Wages are better, schools are being built, water is going through cleaning processes, and value is being added to the found product by cutting the stones and making jewelry in the country where stones are found. This gives more opportunities to the community. We have a pioneering example in Eric Braunwart of Colombia Gemhouse.

A lot more information can be found on the website: www. allianceforanewhumanity.org

In my own experience, we are exploring and developing small mines, searching for golden rutilated quartz associated with hematite. We are working with the state and federal government with registered claims in Bahia, Brazil, paying wages with benefits to the locals. We are creating a preserve all along important headwaters, and introducing permaculture. This will give a new source of wealth to the local people, as eventually stones will be scarce and mining efforts dry up.

Kendra:

Speaking in a more metaphysical perspective, would the removal of precious gems and crystals affect the harmonious energy of the earth?

Brian:

I don't see taking stones from the ground as removing them from the earth. They form in one of the layers of the earth and enter into the biosphere layer of life. My view is that there is a natural evolution. Crystals, gems, and metals are forming as we speak, at great depth. Always have and always will. It is a natural tendency for these elements to come to the surface through orogeny, which literally means the mountain-building process over eons of time. Stones are formed in the deep earth layers and are forced upwards to reach the surface, by uplift and erosion. These energetic materials find their way into the human layer of the planet where they are admired and used, all the way from the early shamans using stones as tools in their practices of astral projection and telepathy, to fashion's high-couture designers who create magnificent jewelry using gems and crystals.

Kendra:

How do gemstones and quartz crystals fit in with the energy of the planet?

Brian:

If one considers the Gaia theory of the living earth, in the minerals—especially gems, quartz, and the solutions involved in the alchemical laboratory of the earth—I may find an analogy with our nervous system. Think of the energy movement and information pathways in fissures, veins, and veinlets distributed all around the earth. We know that silica, which is also in our brains, is conducive to energy movement. It crystallizes in highly energetic veins running through the crust, like a nervous system.

Kendra:

The nervous system in the human body has the purpose of moving information from different types of cells in different parts of the body, in order to access functions for the whole system. Can you comment on the workings of the nervous system for the Gaia model?

Brian:

If I visualize the vast, complex sphere that we live on, I can feel the life of the whole, which includes the biological life. I don't want to venture into "what" the information might be that is carried in the mineralized systems; just knowing that it is all connected, I feel content and feel the wonder of that. I like to imagine the concentrated spots of metals and in all their colors and rich crystal associations distributed in the crust, and the actively-forming base for it all…just makes me go "awe"…"ahh"…

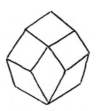

Profiles of Natural Stones

Following are the profiles of a small number of stones, in the order of the visible color spectrum, that are most accessible in stores all over the world. This information was derived from learning about rocks with Brian, the mineral books in the Appendix, and my own knowledge from studying and work-ing with rocks for More then twenty years. Note that the scale of hardness of stones is from 1 (softest) to 10 (hardest). You've read the definition of piezoelectric properties earlier in this chapter.

Purple Quartz • Amethyst

Chemical family: Silicates.

System: Rhombohedral-hexagonal.

Composition: Silica and oxygen, with trace amounts of ferric iron that color it violet.

Place of origin: Brazil, Uruguay, Sri Lanka, Canada, USSR, USA, Africa.

Characteristics: Usually occurs in well-formed crystals; more common in clusters or geodes. Transparent to translucent. Hardness of 7. Piezoelectric properties.

Color: Varies from lavender to deep purple.

History & lore: It was used since early times as a cure for drunkenness and uncontrollable love passion. Influenced by Mars and Jupiter. Astrological sign: Pisces.

Therapeutic and metaphysical information: Stimulates memory, enhancing mental functions. Remedy for insomnia and headaches. Transmutation of energy, purification, ascension. The stone of Saint Germaine and the seventh ray. Balanced between Yin and Yang.

Blue Corundum • Sapphire

Chemical family: Oxides.

System: Hexagonal.

Composition: Oxygen, hydrogen and aluminum.

Place of origin: Africa, Burma, India, Sri Lanka, Thailand, USA.

Characteristics: One of the hardest translucent gemstones, with a hardness of 9. Found as well-formed crystals, or stream gravels.

Color: Blood-red corundum is called ruby. Occurs also in green, pink, orange, yellow and purple. Blue sapphire varies in hue, reaching a desirable vibration of indigo blue. Most commercial stones have been heated to obtain a higher quality of blue.

History & lore: In old England, blue sapphire was used in the treatment of the contagious diseases of the eyes. Ruled by the planets Jupiter and Mercury.

Therapeutic and metaphysical information: Blue sapphire is used to treat mental illnesses, rheumatism, and intestinal disorders in Ayurvedic medicine. Relates to the throat chakra and the pituitary gland. Stimulant of the functions related to the solar plexus.

BLUE BERYL • AQUAMARINE

Chemical family: Silicates.

System: Hexagonal.

Composition: Beryllium, aluminum, silica.

Place of origin: Afghanistan, Brazil, Italy, Nigeria, USA, USSR.

Characteristics: Very hard, 7.5 to 8. Translucent. Occurs with well-formed crystals.

Color: Blue of a light hue, going to a maximum medium blue.

History & lore: Used by high priests in the first century BCE. Aquamarine means seawater. Ruled by the planet Venus.

Therapeutic and metaphysical information: Relates to treating inflammation of the eyes and swollen glands, especially in throat area. Assists in emotional stability and clear communication, cleanser of the throat chakra. Yin influence.

GREEN TOURMALINE

Chemical family: Silicates.

System: Original.

Composition: Complex borosilicate containing magnesium, iron, aluminum, manganese, lithium, silica, oxygen, etc.

Place of origin: Africa, Brazil, Italy, USA, USSR.

Characteristics: Hardness of 7.5 to 8; translucent; piezoelectric properties; well-formed crystals. Complex mineral occurring in all colors of the spectrum.

Color: Green tourmaline varies from light butter-lettuce green to a deep, almost black green.

History & lore: A stone exploited in recent history, after the discovery of the new world, in Brazil. Explorers were looking for emeralds, and thought they had found emerald mines when they discovered green tourmalines. Ruled by the planet Pluto.

Therapeutic and metaphysical information: Immune system and cardiac strengthener. Green tourmaline relates to the herbs that have affinity with healing heart conditions. Yin influence.

GREEN BERYL • EMERALD

Chemical family: Silicates.

System: Hexagonal.

Composition: Beryllium aluminum silicate.

Place of origin: Afghanistan, Africa, Brazil, Columbia, USA.

Characteristics: Very hard but brittle, 7.5 to 8. Transparent, well-formed crystals.

Color: Light to dark green.

History & lore: Attributed to having the prophetic quality of showing the future, through visions seen in the stone. Used for checking the truth in others. Ruled by Venus and Mercury.

Therapeutic and metaphysical information: Valuable for strengthening the spinal column. Stone of general healing energies dealing with issues of manifesting truth. Relates to the heart chakra. Balanced between Yin and Yang.

Yellow Quartz • Citrine

Chemical family: Silicates.

System: Rhombohedral-hexagonal.

Composition: Oxygen, silica and iron hydrates.

Place of origin: Brazil, France, Madagascar, USSR.

Characteristics: Hardness of 7, piezoelectric properties. Transparent; sometimes occurring as well-formed crystals.

Color: Varies from a clear ivory yellow, to yellow, smoky yellow and a rare rich amber gold.

History & lore: Not existent in records to my knowledge.

Therapeutic and metaphysical information: Healing influence for those suffering from asthma. This is a Yang vibrational influence for the solar plexus, helping disperse blocking energies from negative emotions that are keeping the body in a morbid state.

Rutilated Quartz

Chemical family: Quartz: Silicates. Rutile: Oxides.

System: Quartz: Rhombohedral-hexagonal. Rutile: Tetragonal.

Composition: Quartz: Oxygen and silica. Rutile: Oxygen and titanium.

Place of origin: Brazil, Madagascar, Switzerland.

Characteristics: Well-formed quartz crystals containing rutile crystals captured inside their structure. Hardness of 7 for the quartz and of 6 to 6.5 for the rutile crystals. Piezoelectric properties.

Color: Quartz can be clear or smoky. The smoky color is caused by exposure to natural radioactivity. Rutile crystals can occur in different hues of gold, copper, reddish or silvery color.

History & lore: Not existent in records to my knowledge.

Therapeutic and metaphysical information: I have been living with abundant rutilated quartz in my environment for ten years and I have distinctly observed that is has an energizing effect on the nervous system and the solar plexus. Balanced between Yin and Yang. "Helps assimilation of life force, and all nutrients are easier assimilated. Tends to reverse disorders associated with a lowered immune system." - Gurudas.

Orange Topaz • Imperial

Chemical family: Silicates.

System: Orthorhombic.

Composition: Aluminum, iron, hydrogen, oxygen and silica.

Place of origin: Brazil, Siberia.

Characteristics: Hardness of 8, translucent, bright luster; very hard, but brittle. Occurs as well-formed crystals.

Color: Light, medium and deep golden orange, and pinkish orange.

History & lore: This stone has a curious lore of being looked at by seamen for guidance in nights with no moon, to guide their course. Seen as having affinity with the light of the sun, it was used to eliminate fear of the night.

Therapeutic and metaphysical information: Relates to all conditions requiring vitality, warmth, Yang energy. Rejuvenating. Dynamic living symbol for divine love. Ruled by the Sun and Saturn; relates to the solar plexus. Yang influence.

Rose Quartz

Chemical family: Silicates.

System: Hexagonal.

Composition: Oxygen, silica, manganese, titanium.

Place of origin: Brazil, Madagascar, USA.

Characteristics: Hardness of 7, piezoelectric properties. Translucent. Rarely occurs as well-formed crystals. More commonly found in masses. Often included and fractured.

Color: Varies from a clear light to medium pink and milky baby pink.

History & lore: This stone has no recorded history to my knowledge.

Therapeutic and metaphysical information: Relates to feelings and the heart with a tranquilizing effect. It is helpful to balance emotions affecting internal organs. Balanced between Yin and Yang, ruled by the planet Venus.

Red Garnet

Chemical family: Silicates.

System: Isometric.

Composition: Aluminum, calcium magnesium, oxygen, silica.

Place of origin: Brazil, Czechoslovakia, India, USA, Siberia, Africa.

Characteristics: Hardness between 6.5 and 7.5. Translucent to transparent; well-formed isometric crystals.

Color: Varies in all the hues of oranges, reds and reddish browns.

History & lore: Sacred stone of the Native American Indians, Aztecs and other native peoples throughout the world, it was also used in the breastplates of high priests in the Middle Ages. It was used as a protection against the spilling of blood in wars.

Therapeutic and metaphysical information: Red garnet relates to the sacral chakra as a purifying and invigorating influence. Circulatory conditions and sexual ailments; energies of manifestation and strong movement of energy.

RED TOURMALINE

Chemical family: Silicates.

Composition: Complex borosilicates, containing magnesium, iron, aluminum, manganese, lithium, silica, oxygen, etc.

Place of origin: Afghanistan, Brazil, Madagascar, USA.

Characteristics: Hardness of 7.5. Transparent to translucent; piezoelectric properties; well-formed crystals known as rubellite.

Color: Varies from lovely violet pink, to pink-pink and deep red.

History & lore: Not existent in records to my knowledge.

Therapeutic and metaphysical information: Relates to stimulating circulatory movement of the blood and of frequencies merging the sexual with the heart chakra vibrations. Relates to the sacral chakra. Yang.

Smoky Quartz

Chemical family: Silicates.

System: Rhombohedral-hexagonal.

Composition: Silica and oxygen.

Place of origin: Brazil, Scotland, Switzerland, USA.

Characteristics: Occurs as well-formed crystals and in uncrystallized masses. Transparent. Hardness of 7. Piezoelectric properties. The smoky color is caused by exposure to natural radioactivity.

Color: Varies from gray to amber brown and deep brown.

History & lore: Not existent in records to my knowledge.

Therapeutic and metaphysical information: Maintains quality of grounding static energies from all the chakras; balanced Yin and Yang polarities. Relates to the base chakra. Introspection.

Black Tourmaline

Chemical family: Silicates.

System: Trigonal.

Composition: Complex borosilicates containing magnesium, iron, aluminum, manganese, lithium, silica, oxygen, etc.

Place of origin: Brazil, USA.

Characteristics: Hardness of 7.5; piezoelectric properties; well-formed crystals.

Color: Opaque black with a highly lustrous surface.

History & lore: Not existent in records to my knowledge.

Therapeutic and metaphysical information: Used treating those exposed to radiation. Highly absorbent quality, eliminating negative energies. Yang influence.

BLACK JADE

Chemical family: Silicates.

System: Monoclynic.

Composition: Aluminum, iron, silica and sodium.

Place or origin: Australia, Burma, China, USA.

Characteristics: Hardness of 6.5 to 7, crystallized form very rare. Compact and tough. Opaque to translucent. Partially translucent.

Color: Jadeite occurs in all colors including black and white.

History & lore: Considered a sacred stone by different native tribes of the world. Used on the breastplate of the European medieval high priest. Chinese cultures hold jade in high esteem, relating it to longevity, male fertility and kidney-related disorders.

Therapeutic and metaphysical information: A stone of endurance, integrity and equanimity, effecting vibrational influences to all conditions requiring these qualities. Base chakra. Yin and Yang influences.

Diamond

Chemical family: Native element.

System: Isometric.

Composition: Carbon.

Place of origin: Australia, Brazil, Africa, USA, and numerous other countries all over the world.

Characteristics: Hardest mineral on earth, 10. Beautiful octahedron crystals, transparent with high surface luster.

Color: Colorless but also occurring in translucent hues of yellow, blue, green, gray, peach, brown, and black.

History & lore: Regarded as a symbol for invulnerability, the diamond has an extensive history of being ingested for all kinds of purposes and ailments, from removing kidney stones to providing superior strength and good luck. Used as jewelry by the high priests of medieval times. Ruled by Venus and Jupiter. Balanced between Yin and Yang.

Therapeutic and metaphysical information: Manifestation of the perfect balance between energy and matter, it transmits the full spectrum of colors and the totality of light frequencies. It can be used in synergy with all other stones, empowering their specific ray transmission, so it can improve or extend the qualities of a stone where the quality is not optimum. The same as the quartz crystal, the diamond can be used in every way with all synergies, but it carries a warmer energy than quartz, which is cooling.

CLEAR QUARTZ

Chemical family: Silicates.

System: Rhombohedral-hexagonal.

Composition: Silica and oxygen.

Place of origin: All over the world.

Characteristics: Occurs as well-formed crystals and in uncrystallized masses. Transparent to translucent. Hardness of 7. Piezoelectric properties.

Color: Colorless.

History & lore: Used as a sacred object by shamans of many native peoples all over the world. Relates to the element silver and to the moon.

Therapeutic and metaphysical information: Like the diamond, clear quartz transmits the full spectrum and can be used in any synergy. Mainly used as a transducer and recorder of energy. Please refer to the beginning of this chapter. Balanced between Yin and Yang.

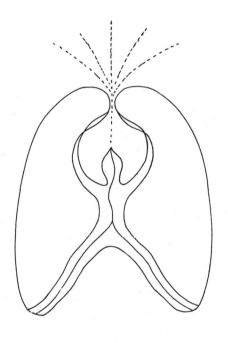

Energy moves through body with intention

PART THREE

Vibrational Healing

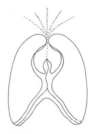

O deep rays of indigo blue,
Bring me in devotion's hours
New found fragrance in brain-flowers
Sweeping all brown leaves away.
~Roland Hunt

Vibrational Healing

When we go on a nature walk, spend a day at the beach or go camping for a number of days, something happens that is more than taking time out to relax away from the intense rhythms of our lives. By merging with our physical environment in nature, we feel expanded and grounded. We become harmonized; the different energetic layers of our being, mind, body and emotions develop a balanced strength that functions more efficiently to support our lives here on earth.

The time has come when metaphysical and scientific thought can work together. We are living a time of integration, as we complete a cycle of focused specialization. When science unites with its "opposite," metaphysics and spirituality, creating wholeness, we will live to experience what seemed to be impossible answers to many crucial questions about life. Many scientists and doctors are now expressing and working with recognition of a more holistic approach in understanding life and medicine.

Elementals

Let's consider the term "elementals," in this context, as "small, organized units performing a function, that form the different unified fields of energy invested in the creation of our bio-dynamic physical bodies." These can be a cell or a group of cells, an organ, and finally the connected whole of our complex physical bodies. Our physical bodies also contain energetics that come from different intangible vibrational fields, interfacing and merging with our physical cells. In a simplistic way, we can point out the mental, emotional, etherical, and even more refined energies that some call causal fields. So, these elementals are invested in the "project" that is our individual selves.

Our communication with our elementals is done from the more subtle layers of thought and emotion, and these more subtle perceptions lead to choices, attitudes. If we feel happy, grateful and blessed, we are living… If we are sad, fearful and depressed, we are dying. These are the messages we transmit to our elementals, living in our physical bodies. When we give this message that we are dying, then they begin to long for their place of origin, nature, the matrix that they came from. This opens the door for other forms of life, either living within or outside our bodies, that are the breakdown and recycling crew: the bacteria, viruses, fungus, and other microorganisms whose job is to disassemble systems; and that is how disease can be created in the body. But as all of life is in a constant state of flux, with a pattern that contracts and expands, turning on and turning off, pulsating in a constant rhythm, our message to the elementals can fluctuate between short or long waves of time. This is how we can recuperate fast, or have a longer period of illness—even so long as to lead to the complete disassembly of the physical self, death. These movements are unconscious or conscious, depending on the evolutionary stage of each soul.

The elementals that have invested together in the creation of our physical bodies have the mission to organize life. The other microorganisms that I called the breakdown crew disassemble, take systems apart.

So…by understanding these concepts, what can we do that could help our healing using vibrational influences?

Remembering that when we seem to want to "give up" on our state of balance, and we give the message to the elementals that we are dying, they long to be released to the greater organism that they came from, the matrix, earth. The first thing is to become conscious of this process, so we can make choices that will result in changes influencing our bodies to go back to a state of balance or health. By using natural elements, powerful influences that are highly energetic life, we can choose to realize useful changes.

Let's look at our doors of perception, the doorways between the inner and the outer worlds, our physical senses. It is through these doorways that we can use the powerful influence of natural elements. Here lies a world of possibilities for harmonizing the different fields of energy living in our physical bodies, creating balance and health.

The Senses and Natural Elements

The whole universe is made up of vibrations. The physical world is made of natural systems that arc interconnected. Natural elements link up to our senses. Aromatic material links to smell, light and color link to vision. Edible nature links to taste, texture and temperature link to touch, sound links to hearing. This is the essential fabric of our natural world, our laboratory of co-creation. So much is possible in creative endeavors with healing, if one has a clear mind and a focused intent.

At the end of this section you will find a correspondence chart. I list the suggested relationship of chakras and body systems to color, stone, essential oils and sound, for creating synergies for use in vibrational healing. Here also is inspiration for meditations and procedures empowering the basic and elemental sensorial experience.

HEARING

Not only is everything pulsating in the universe in an endless rhythm, but also this pulse expresses a "resonance" that can be felt and sometimes heard. Above all, sound is the origin of all manifestations. Many creation stories and mystery schools refer to this. In the West we know the common phrase from the Bible, "In the beginning was the word," (John, 1:1)

Sound permeates and forms all things, so let's take a look at the nature of sound and explore how to use it in vibrational healing.

Frequency, Resonance and Entrainment

Resonance is the frequency or wavelength in which energies, such as colors from the spectrum as well as sound, pulsate. Each one of our different elementals, or organized fields of energy, is vibrating at its own particular rate. Together, the total organism is created with its particular vibratory rate. When imbalances happen, energetic units that are working for a particular function, an organ for example, can go out of tune. By using a strong influence—for instance, the human voice, or a crystal singing bowl, which can emit powerful resonance—one can get the unified field of energy that is out of tune, to "entrain" with the more powerful influence and pulsate together. Entrainment is about synchronization; a less-powerful vibration will "follow" the influence of a more powerful one, and their rhythms will synchronize. After some time the weaker one will remember its own harmonic rate and stabilize its own harmony.

The best way to harmonize the body energy fields is to use the vocal cords of the human voice. In the correspondence chart there are the suggestions for toning all the vowels using the notes of the musical scale, Do, Re, Mi, Fa, So, La, Ti, Do.

Quartz Crystal Singing Bowls

The crystal bowls are produced by the computer industry; they are made from fused quartz-crystal sand, creating a glass that offers tremendous heat resistance. The computer industry uses them to grow the silicon crystal chips used in computers that have to be created in heat up to 4,200 degrees Fahrenheit.

People selling these crystal bowls organize them to present the different notes of the musical scale, which correspond to the different chakras. (See correspondence chart.) I have a set of these crystal bowls; each one resonates with a different frequency.

The song of the crystal bowls can help harmonize the different energy fields pulsating in the human body, creating an overall balance. It is easy to feel their influence.

The highly-acclaimed musician Stephen Halpern has recorded the sound of the crystal bowls in his musical work "Crystal Suite." Stephen said: "In all my work with acoustic and electronic instruments, including Japanese and Tibetan bowls, these quartz bowls represent a unique and extraordinary resource."

Many sound therapists all around the world are using crystal bowls. Look for resources in the Appendix.

OLFACTORY

Nothing is more compelling to the sense of smell than the influence of aromatic plants. Aromatic plants create a special link between mind and body, relaxation and sensuality. One can be delighted in the colors expressed by flowers, and color can modify mood, directing the mind to relaxation or otherwise. However, when one smells a scent, one can feel an instantaneous reaction in the body. Lungs will breathe deeper, the heart can beat faster or slower; the brain can awake to memories, bringing beads of perspiration to the skin, and surprising emotions can surface causing all kinds of reactions in the body. Sweet-smelling nature has always guided us to the exuberance of our sensual core, bringing us true feelings of well-being and spontaneous sexuality. This guidance can create a seed for health and happiness.

Association and Relationship

Together, a certain smell and a particular experience are recorded in our brain's emotional archive. When experience stimulates a certain emotion, a feeling remains on record in the brain. Thoughts can be lost, but feelings can stay with the precision of a flawless operation. The feeling is in direct relationship to memory. Memory is a mechanism that is biologically set up to operate with the senses. One will remember a scene that was once viewed, a taste that was once experienced, a touch that was once felt, a sound that was once heard, but the most direct, primal and powerful—however elusive—sense, linking to memory, is certainly the smell.

The awakening of the smell experience from memory is often startling and extraordinary. This provides tremendous potential for therapies involving harmonization of emotional and mental states, which can extend to heal ill conditions in the body.

In my experience of working with *therapy by aroma*, I have been continuously surprised to find constant common denominators, conditions needed in so many circumstances. Following are the primary ones:

1. A smell provides an opportunity for mental focus.
2. A smell provides a support system in times of crisis, distress, and everyday stress.
3. A smell links an individual's awareness of the body/ mind connection.

The relationship between smell and memory holds a tremendous potential for a healer or therapist working with emotional and mental states of the individual. The limbic system, the area of the brain processing memory and emotion, is also where the cells that process the information coming from the nerve endings connecting to the olfactory bulb are located. Memory and emotion are not associated with odor processing by chance. We need information from our sense of smell to survive. One simple example is detecting a decomposing smell on a portion of food prior to eating it. From that information comes the the decision to discard the food. If our sense of smell were not functioning properly, we could eat food that would make us sick. Next time the same type of food is served, unconsciously our "smell brain" will process the memory of the previous smell and automatically do a comparison to the present one. This is one example of the myriads of subtle ways that we ordinarily use odor/memory processing. Most times this happens unconsciously.

If one desires to use this function consciously, as an aid in therapies, there are numerous ways to proceed. One general way is to use a positive association in order to achieve a certain result. Hospitals frequently give a child in the operating room the smell of chocolate, to distract its fear by creating a feeling with a positive association.

Besides the association of smell with a past or present experience, there is the relationship of smell with the unified field of energy.

A unified field of energy can be defined as organized matter performing functions within a unit: a cell, an organism such as our bodies, plants, animals, minerals; all natural elements and manmade systems also—a computer, a car, an iPod. These unified fields of energy contain a number of interconnecting layers, all the way from cells and organs to electromagnetic and subtler mechanisms. These organized forms enable our systems to link up within themselves, and to the energies moving in the greater planetary organism that supports all life here, the earth.

Let's consider the relationship between the unified field of energy of a certain plant, and the unified field of energy of an individual. The plant is specialized. Its system has codes of information that are sophisticated messages from many levels and nuances of its life, and will, like a drop of water to the sea, naturally reach out for links to other unified fields of energy. A subtle communication is engaged between a plant and a human being, linking up from the senses to functions in the brain, including memory and emotion.

An individual will retain information from seeing colors and shapes of this plant and its parts, from feeling its leaves and flowers, trunk and stem. Sounds from the plants are not captured in the scope of the perceptible notes in our hearing, yet are absorbed by more subtle mechanisms of our audition. (See *The Secret Life of Plants*, by Tompkins and Bird). Plants are tasted and eaten and will deliver nutritional and vibrational elements that link to our systems. If the plant is aromatic, its aromatic molecules will link directly to our brain through the olfactory bulb, delivering information that creates records for further use in myriad of links, which can have therapeutic effects on body, mind and emotion.

Aromatic plants are highly specialized healers from the plant kingdom. Not only do they ignite certain effects in our bodies, but they also create a record in the smell brain to be accessed later, as they perform the effect. These effects can be organized into a general performance, as well as a more specific and personal nuance having to do with the relationship between the fields in consideration. The general performance of essential oils has been observed, understood and defined scientifically; either sedation or stimulation of our bodies' metabolism. As the effect takes place, transference of information between neurons either slows down or speeds up. This is the foundation of aromatherapy; the general physical effects that are known about essential oils and their aromas on our metabolism. Functions in the brain also utilize smell to ignite automatic logic and understanding, in order for the individual to access decision-making processes regarding protection, direction, rejection and attraction.

Other considerations regarding relationship on the level of the earth and her natural systems, including ourselves, are in the composition of an essential oil. There are elements of intricate complexity to consider, for they coordinate innumerable amounts of changeable information coming from the energies that are in constant flux: the seasons, the weather, the temperature, the soil, the amount of water from rainfall, the intensity of the sun. All the mutable elements communicate a sort of planetary mood, to be registered specially in the molecules that we call trace elements, linking to our unified field. These are the mutable parts of an aromatic composition, that which has the latest and more dynamic links to the greater organism, our matrix, the earth. Those are precisely the parts of the composition of an essential oil that, taken to the lab to be developed for commercial use, must be "purified," or rather stripped out, because they are too mutable to be replicated in the composition of a formula.

Aromatherapists speak of plant-source, first-distillation, genuine essential oils as having "life force"; the ancient Egyptians spoke of aromatic plants as being "life giving." I find a correlation between this way of thinking and the mutable part of the composition of an essential oil, the trace elements. I think of this as nature's artistic endeavor, like a symbolic language, speaking of mysteries that are beyond the range of basic comprehension. Its qualities have definitions equal to what we define as spirit.... a volatile, intangible, yet powerful, ephemeral presence that connects us to the source of life.

What happens between people and plants has always left me in a state of awe. How did an early healer, a primitive shaman, get the information that led to his knowledge regarding specific uses of his plants? Now that we have vast amounts of information that has been passed down through many time periods and societies, the first information, going right along and growing with more developing discoveries, remains as the original thought about the plant, its history. All plant mythology is a story between God and man. As scientists investigate what has been found in earlier times, we create a synergy of thought about the therapeutics of plants; a body of knowledge is formed between lore and science. My idea is that intuition played an important role in the beginning of this knowledge. In Brazil, I have experienced among healers and shamans the concept that the divine appoints someone. From there on, this individual holds a responsibility within his society, to serve and to heal and to link minds to a greater knowledge about life.

Flower Power

Primarily the oils of the flowers, specially the steam-distilled ones—rose, orange blossoms (neroli), and lavender—are my favorite for *therapy by aroma*. Flowers are heart openers. Consider the many energetic fields that merge into the chakras. Chakras are the gateways from and to the different levels of our unified fields of energy. Flower oils have the power to open the chakras, creating an energetic movement that directs a flow with the aromatic message from the oil to the different systems in the body. This action connects the body to the matrix, the earth, with the use of this natural element. Rose creates a flow from the heart to the circulatory system, and from there to all the other systems in the body, working to eliminate blocks—physical, emotional, etc…and orange blossom creates a flow from the heart to the nervous system, instilling a powerful sedative effect. So, by only the smell itself, it can vibrationally help someone to slow cardiac contractions and even avoid a heart attack. Both these oils can be ingested (See see Medical Aromatherapy: Making Teas), but they will also work vibrationally just by smelling them. Lavender is a purifier, and smelling it clears the lungs and gives comfort to the whole system.

Smell alone will stop stressful mental chatter. One cannot smell and think at the same time. In smelling, one has to focus, giving a little break to the never-ending thoughts. This is spontaneously a anti-stress activity.

Smell and Imagery

Essential oils can empower your work with imagery, if you begin to perceive the aromatic molecules as energy that transforms you in the same way that the invisible energies from the visualized images you create can also make you feel calmer or more energized. One can use an essential oil to bring one's mind power into a more tangible form. This is because the invisible but tangible element of the essential oils, the smell, will serve as a bridge between the intangible reality of one's visualized image, and the ordinary palpable reality of the aromatic molecules from the essential oils.

So if visualization has always been an important element in mind power, imagine how much more powerful it becomes in synergy with an aroma. You can use the field of energy created by images + aromatic molecules to transmit desired changes to yourself or somebody else. One has to become aware of the physical and the nonphysical at the same time, and focus on that union with the intention of performing transformation and enabling the change of consciousness in different energy fields of the body.

In co-creating with the invisible energy of the oils, holding a clear intention and carrying a bond for further interactions, subliminally you will be receiving information from the codes in the molecules themselves, which all proceed from the greater living organism, the earth.

THERAPY BY AROMA

The following real-life stories illustrate a few of the ways in which therapies by aroma can be helpful.

Marty Winn

General Contractor in his late thirties, Sebastopol, California.

Kendra: Marty had a pre-existing heart condition from a previous car accident. I visited him in the hospital after a second accident. A school bus had collided with his sports car, fracturing eight of his ribs, breaking his femur in six pieces, crushing his kneecap and ankle, and splitting his tibia lengthwise. He had two severe skull fractures and his collarbone and sternoclavicular and rotator cuff joints were broken. Marty was in traction and on morphine when I came in to visit him at the beginning of his second week in the hospital. This man was in serious trouble; a big, strong guy who could normally lift 300 lbs. over his head with no trouble at all, now lay in the hospital bed unable to lift his own arm, waiting for the life-or-death decision of his second surgery.

The hospital personnel were so intensely busy trying to fix his body, that I felt they had forgotten Marty altogether. From my perspective, I knew immediately he desperately needed help getting his mind to focus and his emotions to heal, as importantly as his body.

In his situation he did not need any kind of explanation about the therapy I was about to do with him, because his mind was saturated with life-or-death issues and his body was in such bad shape that teaching seemed absolutely inappropriate. A wordless aromatic experience was all I perceived was necessary to address his emotional situation, and I used a strongly sedative blend made from rose otto, neroli and lavender placed inside an Aromajewel hanging from the metal apparatus just above his nose.

Marty: As I was absolutely helpless, lying there wondering if I was going to live or die, I was looking for emotional contact. I was not getting that in the hospital. I remember the aromatic smell. First I kind of liked it, but after a while I had a judgment. This was not some kind of wild splash or something!

I knew it was essential oils and I didn't believe in therapeutic properties or anything. I think my emotional bond with Kendra made me trust something that normally I would have thought to be off the wall and disconnected with what was going on.

The fragrance was extremely different. All of sudden there was a whole new world I could be in and exit my body. Now I was getting something for me. It was like an escape. Lying there with the TV on, I was in a daze from all the drugs, held together by stitches and pins, connected to hoses and tubes, and I needed another space to be in. With this little, fragrant crystal I could close my eyes, take great deep breaths and smell this aroma that was putting me in a euphoric state. Made me feel like I could leave my body, and heightened my ability to be able to check my mind out from the pain and check into a state where I was emotionally aware without being emotional. I felt my self inside saying, "I am all right, I am going to be O.K." This gave me a positive dimension; it strengthened my emotions enough to face surgery, and as a result, my recovery was a lot faster than expected. I had that crystal with me until after I went home. It supported me emotionally much more than anything or anybody. I could lie there, cover my face, breathe deep and go into another world. It was better than drugs or even prayers. I would come back energized and ready to repair my body. I was rather surprised at what I received in this little piece of jewelry.

Carla Dykes

Young mother in her twenties, Sebastopol, California.

Kendra: Carla had a physical condition arising from the result of open-heart surgery when she was five years old. Her surgery had severed nerves and she had no sensation in her left breast. She was pregnant, with her second baby due to be born any minute and still had her first baby, less than two years old, nursing regularly. Her nursing with the first child had some difficulty, especially emotional because she could not feel the let-down reflex in one of her breasts and worried that her baby was not getting enough milk. This created a fear-based block that was building with the second child coming, since there was a good chance she would be nursing two babies at once for a while.

When I saw Carla we had a session in which we discussed this type of therapy using aromas to help her remove the mental/emotional block. Together we created visual imagery to represent an opening in the energy of the block, relaxing mind and body. She focused on the imagery while smelling the aroma of Turkish rose otto that I was applying on her breast through massage. We did this a few times, and in between sessions I left with her the aromatic crystal with the same smell for her to meditate and continue the influence in between sessions.

Carla: This therapy using an aroma was beneficial to me in terms of comforting me in a stressful time, helping relax the fear. This initiated a process in me so a change was possible. It gave me an open perspective in how I can grow in my ability to trust alternative therapies for my healing. I felt the crystal broaden the spectrum of the healing. The stone and plant oil combination connected me to a greater natural support system in a time when I needed that. I used the aroma to meditate and that was very healing.

Dr. David Kent

An M.D. anesthesiologist in his fifties, Santa Rosa, California.

Kendra: Dr. Kent had a serious pelvic fracture from a rollerblading accident. Being familiar with the hospital environment, he was comfortable and knew the people attending him. His surgery was successful and he and his surgeon were pretty happy with the results. When I came to visit him, he was in the rehabilitation unit and had developed a blood clot in his right leg, which had a risk of migrating to his lungs, causing cardiac function and respiratory problems. He is a strong, active man and was hoping for his maximum recovery.

It was obvious his main emotional issue was accepting his "soaking" period in bed, without being able to do much and not knowing how long he would be there. There was apprehension and nervousness regarding what the outcome would be. My input with Dr. Kent was purely intuitive. I felt that his condition was Yin, arising from a situation when he was fast-moving and had a violent halt. The blood clot developed some days after the surgery. To me this seemed to match the slowing of movement, causing the Yin condition, now in his blood circulation. I decided to bring him a blood-colored Aromajewel, a red tourmaline with purple hues with Chinese ginger oil in it, which created a strong Yang influence for his electromagnetic field with the intention to focus on creating balance. I told him to use the synergy, visualizing the Yin/Yang balance and the dissolving of the clot.

Dr. Kent: Kendra came to visit at a time when I was waiting for the blood to thin to avoid further complication with the blood clot that had developed after the accident. There was not much I could do but just lie there with very little exercise and wait. She loaned me a heart-shaped pendant with ginger oil in it. I did get in trouble shortly after her visit, as the blood clot broke loose and I went to the intensive care unit for a couple of days. Gradually I improved and eventually got out of the hospital, which I ended up staying in for a total of four weeks.

I wore the aromatic stone with the ginger oil most of the time while in the hospital. What I felt with that was an energizing, yet gentle, positive, psychological feeling. It was not like having perfume under my nose, but it was there and I could notice it and be aware of it and get a waft from it once in a while. It helped me focus on feeling positive, by bringing my attention and my awareness to the healing process, as a reminder to put some energy into healing. It frequently reminded me to focus on this positive aspect. I did feel that it was a positive, energetic thing and not a hypnotizing, passive or sleep-inducing thing. When I was alone, it kept bringing my attention back to my body healing, by using my own energy.

Something that also happened, is that the ginger smell made a memory pop up of a time, years before, when I was traveling in New Guinea with three good friends and we went hiking where there were ginger flowers growing along the trails. This was a very happy time of my life, when I was exploring this vibrant and alive jungle environment, doing a lot of athletic and energetic climbing. At a time when I was in a hospital bed, I had this memory association with exercise and the reddish purple ginger flowers of New Guinea. A very strong positive feeling.

Angela Peroba

A reporter in her thirties, Salvador, Bahia, Brazil.

Kendra: Angela had been trying to conceive a child for a number of years, and she and her husband had already done several different tests and treatments. It was discovered she had a small obstruction in one of her fallopian tubes but this was not a probable reason for her inability to conceive. She was seeing a psychotherapist at the time I saw her, and she was eager to try everything available that might have a chance of helping her. I spoke to her about psycho-aromatherapy and she wanted to try aromas. We scheduled an appointment and I brought a calming oil with me, the absolute of orange blossom. First we had a conversation and she told me the situation in detail. Soon I noticed that she was trying to help her body with her mind but as she went into more and more concepts, she would churn and churn large amounts of stress-forming material. I knew this session had to focus on only body and scent, leaving the mind with just the image she needed to associate to the smell of orange blossoms. I gave her a full-body massage, with the intent of our decision in mutual focus. It was pretty obvious to me as I started that the problem in her body was fear-based tension, developed to such a extent that her reproductive function was shutting down. If only she could get herself to relax, truly she would conceive. I left her with an Aromajewel, some more neroli oil, and massage oil with the same aroma in more diluted form for her to use daily on her abdomen as she did a little meditation, keeping the focus of what we had registered at the time of the therapy. After our treatment she felt very optimistic and continued searching for more help from metaphysical, spiritual and traditional medicine methods. Less than two months later I received a letter from her, giving me the happy news of her first pregnancy.

Angela: I feel something opened with our aroma work. I thank you again. I feel that this experience with the aromatherapy is somehow difficult to separate what happened, in my body, emotions and mind. When I reflect on it, what becomes clear is that this therapy via aroma worked its way in me in a very effective way that I want to call Global. Principally it provided me a trust that my searching was going to succeed. With the orange blossom I felt my trust growing as if I was being showered with the scent of happiness. Next to the trust, I felt a synchronicity, with more serenity between my internal and external movements. Without a doubt, the aromatherapy participated effectively and in a holistic way with the traditional medicine that I engaged in shortly afterwards.

Facts concerning the sense of smell

The sense of smell can stimulate alertness, memory, learning, sensitivity, self-esteem, awareness of wholeness, receptivity to information, elimination of stress, and reproductive system functions.

- Sexual excitement increases olfactory capacity.
- Olfactory deprivation can contribute to Alzheimer's disease and madness.
- Sensory deprivation can mutate genetic codes.
- A child can identify the mother by smell and vice-versa.
- One may not be able to relax in an environment with unfamiliar smells.
- The smell of body odors is affected by diet.
- Stress, habitual stressful thoughts and other emotional conditions modify body odor.
- Some of male and female attraction is processed via smell.
- Pheromones, chemicals detected in sweat, urine, and feces, also exist in the vomenal nasal organ and are molecules containing messages that trigger sexual behavior.
- Smell, being processed by the right brain, stimulates the feeling center.

Body Odor Meditation

This is an exercise that will heighten your awareness of self and stimulate conscious holistic self-learning and acceptance, giving you a sense of internal harmony and peace. To do it, you need to be ready for a lesson of surrender, humility, fear-facing and concentration. It is done in a bathtub in a silent and dim environment, and you will need to have a naturally sweaty body with the absence of any body care products. You can do it after a busy working day, after working out, or after a couple of days without bathing.

Procedure: Center yourself and calm down your thinking process. Direct focus on yourself and your breathing pattern. Fill the bathtub with water as hot as you can stand it. If it is winter make sure the bathroom is warm. Slowly place yourself only up to your waist in the water. Sit comfortably and soon you should begin to sweat noticeably. Concentrate on the perception of positive feelings you have had about yourself. Take time with yourself, emptying the mind and just feeling your body and emotions. Soon you will begin to feel surrounded by your own body smell. Focus on placing no judgment and relax into it, in equanimity. Develop the situation to the point that you are breathing freely and enjoyably, with the focus on your own body odor surrounding you. When you feel that you have experienced the totality of this encounter with self, you can bathe and get out of the experience. Notice what happens in your relationship with your self in the days that follow this experience.

SIGHT

The influence of natural elements through the doorways to the sense of sight relies on light and color.

Turn to the chart at the end of this section to see the relationship of each body system to its beneficial color. The correspondence on the chart relates to the chakras, which are to be understood here as the pulsation that transmits the color of the spectrum to the physical body. Let's take the example of the solar plexus, related to the digestive system. In order to use light to capture the yellow/gold ray of the spectrum for vibrational healing, one can use a quartz crystal. Choose a crystal that has good clarity and sharp edges with smooth faces. This crystal has to be positioned in a good angle in relationship to strong sunlight. Natural sunlight, as it diffracts in the crystal, will create a rainbow that can be used to direct that particular color of the ray directly to the iris of the person wanting a certain color to energize a specific system.

Also, for great enjoyment one can infuse the system through the eyes with all the colors of the rainbow, using natural sunlight. This will require two people sharing this procedure, as the one receiving the color through the iris will have to lie down and relax, looking at the diffraction and directing the desired ray of the light, while the other will have to hold the crystal in the sunlight and work at the achieving the perfect angle for the best rainbow light, positioning the colors into the iris of the partner. This procedure is safe, as the diffracted colors of the rainbow light is a small light, much less than 10 percent of the actual sunlight. One should not look at the sunlight, but at the diffracted rainbow light coming out of the crystal.

Remember that strong lights, such as laser lights that people use for color therapy, would be harmful to the eyes and to be avoided by all means. This suggestion is only for natural rainbow light through the diffraction from a quartz crystal. One could use a glass crystal and that would not be harmful to the eyes, but the difference is that quartz crystal has an organized structure from an energy field that transmits the colors through its own lattice of a natural system matrix. Glass is an amorphous, unstructured medium made from fused quartz sand.

I have done this procedure for many, many years and I always use one of my Stargems crystals as they have an extraordinary optical quality and sharpness of angles. As this provides a very different experience, I have seen many people be tremendously and positively affected by it, almost to a sentimental point, as if they were given a rainbow to swim in.

Vibrant sunrises and sunsets are very beneficial for empowering the solar and sacral chakras affecting the urinary system and the sexual organs.

Taste

Minerals break down into soil, releasing all their elements, and the plants take them into their bodies and combine these elements and metals that were once rocks into a system with organic molecules. We eat the plants, absorbing the metals and trace elements that are so important in the biological functions of our bodies. We receive the nourishment from the elements ingested and we also receive informational codes that are vibrational and that are being transmitted through-out all the kingdoms of nature, uniting and connecting us to the full cycle that is the continuous movement of life. When we die, all the elements or elementals that were invested into our bodies go back to our matrix, the earth, and go through all the kingdoms again—physical, as well as vibrational.

Likewise, as the colored stones, flowers, fruit, vegetables and all the edible green part of nature are colored by the minerals that they absorb from the soil to create their bodies. A beet is rich in iron, as is a red tourmaline or garnet. The color of deep red will add to the richness of our blood, also aiding the circulation, sexual organs, and the urinary system, as we see in the correspondence chart.

Taste is divided into different experiences; sweet, sour, bitter and salty. These different experiences in taste send us signals from our taste buds about what is necessary to our systems. Have you ever wondered why, in a whole table full of differ-ent dishes, you don't seem to find what you are craving? Your taste buds know. They work at organizing what is necessary for ingestion. If you had an episode of food poisoning one night, you will know what not to eat the following morning, and your body will tell you what to eat that feels right on the following day. Of course, in modern life, the seduction of consumer products has a way to manipulate desire and taste buds in a much more sophisticated way than was originally intended by nature.

Exercise:

Here is a nice procedure to infuse the system with a color that relates to taste for vibrational healing. Choose a food in the color group that relates to the body system you are working to influence. Eat the food with that color, and visualizing the same color as you hold the intent of harmonizing that system or organ, lie down to digest what you ingested, covering yourself with a cloth in that same color. Example: For an influence on the heart use a green sheet and a green salad, visualizing the rich green one sees in nature. For an even stronger influence, drop rose or orange blossom oil on a handkerchief, and tone the vocal cords with all the vowels in the note of Fa.

Touch

Again, as there is nothing as good at influencing the gateway to hearing than the human voice, there is nothing that can affect the physical body like the human touch. This can speak for all the different modalities of massage that humans have done since the beginning of all times. Some touch deeply enough to address the different muscle groups, ligaments and nerve endings, and some touch gently, such as the laying on of hands, Reiki, and other modalities affecting the more subtle levels of the human body, the more electric and ethereal energy fields.

In 1996, at a workshop in the Swiss Alps called *Dreaming the Dance of the Senses*, I gathered a dozen people to have experiences with exercises to influence the different senses. We used Stargems for creating rainbows and experiencing the different colors of the spectrum going into the iris, we had our eyes closed in meditation to experience scent and taste, quartz crystal singing bowls for hearing, and for the sense of touch we had different-textured objects: sea sponges, smooth sculpted stones in different shapes, small grains, sharp metals, etc…These objects were lying in a basin of water at body temperature, and we would put our hands in the water to experience the different textures and thermal feelings received by the nerve endings in our hands. We used this as a sensorial meditation, quieting the mind of thoughts and substituting the sensation of touch. We ended the session with a type of contact improvisation dance, using our bodies for a light touch exploration of shape and temperature, with eyes closed. The bodies become a human landscape, and this is done as a sensorial meditation, with a focused intent not to have a sexual arousal, as that would change the experience completely. This is a unique form of meditation that can train focus and intent in a very powerful way.

As we are talking about experiences with the sense of touch here, I want to share that I have experienced a type of massage called Watsu (Water+Shiatsu) that was developed in 1980 by Harold Dull in Harbin Hot Springs, Middletown, California. Watsu is a form of bodywork done in a shallow pool at body temperature. This type of massage stretches ligaments and addresses pressure points to release blocks. There is a lot that can be done on a floating body with joints suspended in the water, which cannot be done on a massage table. I am writing about my experience with Watsu here because it gave me an opportunity to return in feeling to a primal state of the first feelings of touch, like the first experience of the skin being formed in the womb. Watsu is now offered around the world in many different spas and with practitioners and some practitioners have developed a "water dance" style that has a free-flowing technique.

Full-body Clay Mask

For a simple procedure with touch and thermal stimulation, you can do a full-body clay mask at home.

You will need a bowl where you can mix the clay of your choice (see pages 112–113) in water; depending on your body size you will need approximately 24 ounces of clay. You want a thick pack that will take some time to dry completely. Cover the body completely, and the face as well. Cover the body with a lightweight cloth for the drying process. Meditate on the sensation, your breath, and the openness to accept the grounding influence of the earth on your skin. After this procedure you shower, and moisturize the body with oils or lotion.

In addition, you can also choose the corresponding essential oil from the chart addressing the body system or part that you want to influence. You can use all the other elements on the chart or not; use this as well for pleasure and purification, using your creative imagination.

VIBRATIONAL HEALING
CORRESPONDENCE CHART

Chakra	Color	Stone	Essential Oil	Sound	Body System or Organ
base	black, brown, red	black tourmaline, black jade, garnet, red tourmaline, smoky quartz	frankincense, myrrh, patchouli, vetiver	toning of all vowels in DO	blood circulation, gonads
sacral	red, orange,	garnet, imperial topaz, red tourmaline, rose quartz	jasmine, rose, sandalwood, ylang ylang	toning of all vowels in RE	sexual organs, urinary system
solar plexus	yellow, gold	citrine, rutilated quartz, golden beryl	basil, clary sage, lemon, orange blossom	toning of all vowels in MI	digestive system, stomach, liver, adrenal glands
heart	green, pink	emerald, green tourmaline, pink tourmaline, rose quartz	bergamot, geranium, orange blossom, rose	toning of all vowels in FA	circulatory system, heart, thymus gland
throat	light and medium blue, silver	aquamarine, blue tourmaline, silver	all chamomiles, orange blossom (neroli)	toning of all vowels in SO	respiratory system, lungs, thyroid gland
third eye	lavender, deep blue, indigo	deep blue tourmalines, sapphire, amethyst	lavender, rosemary	toning of all vowels in LA	nervous system, pituitary gland
crown	violet, gold, white	amethyst, diamond, gold	frankincense, jasmine, lavender, sandalwood	toning of all vowels in TI and high DO	central nervous system, pineal gland

Appendix

Suggested Reading

Aromatherapy & Essential Oils

Aftel, Mandy.
Essence and Alchemy. North Point Press, 2001.

Catty, Suzanne.
Hydrosols: The Next Aromatherapy. Healing Arts Press, 2000.

Cunningham, Scott.
Magical Aromatherapy. Llewellyn Publications, 1989.

Damian, Peter and Kate.
Aromatherapy: Scent and Psyche. Inner Traditions, 1995.

Davis, Patricia.
Aromatherapy: An A to Z. Saffron Walden, 1988.
Subtle Aromatherapy. Daniel, 1991.

England, Allison.
Aromatherapy for Mother and Baby. Healing Arts Press, 1994.

Fawcett, Margaret, R.M.
Aromatherapy for Pregnancy and Childbirth. Penguin, 1993.

Franchomme, P. and Pénoël, D.
L'aromatherapie exactment. Roger Jollois, 1990.

Gattefossé, Rene-Maurice.
Gattefossé's Aromatherapy. C.W. Daniel, 1993.

Grace, Kendra.
Aromatherapy Pocketbook. Llewellyn Publications, 1999.

Green, Mindy, and Keville, Katty.
Aromatherapy: A Complete Guide to the Healing Art. Crossing Press, 1995.

Gunter, Ernest.
The Essential Oils, 6 volumes. D. Van Nostrand, 1948-1952.

Lavabre, Marcel.
Aromatherapy Workbook. Healing Arts Press, 1990.

Lawless, Julia.
The Encyclopedia of Essential Oils. Element, 1992.
The Illustrated Encyclopedia of Essential Oils. Element, 1995.
Aromatherapy and the Mind. Thorson, 1994.

Leigh, Ixchel.
Aromatic Alchemy. Mansion Publishing, 2001.

Lind, Eva Marie.
Aromatiques. Soma Publishing, 2002.

Maury, M. Marguerite.
Maury's Guide to Aromatherapy. Daniel, 1988.

Miller, Light and Bryan.
Ayurveda and Aromatherapy. Lotus Light, 1996.

Mojay, Gabriel.
Aromatherapy for Healing the Spirit. Healing Arts Press, 1997.

Price, Shirley.
Practical Aromatherapy. Thorsons, 1983.
Aromatherapy for Health Professionals. Churchill Livingston, 1995.

Rose, Jeanne.
The Aromatherapy Book. North Atlantic Books, 1992.

Rose, Jeanne, and Earle, Susan, Eds.
The World of Aromatherapy. Frog. Ltd., 1996.

Schnaubelt, Kurt, Ph.D.
Advanced Aromatherapy. Inner Traditions, 1997.
Medical Aromatherapy. Frog, Ltd., 1999.

Tisserand, Maggie.
Aromatherapy for Women. Thorsons, 1985.

Tisserand, Robert.
The Art of Aromatherapy. Inner Traditions, 1977.

The E.O. Safety Data Manual. Tisserand Aromatherapy Institute, 1990.

Valnet, Jean, Duraffour, and Lapraz, Jean Claude.
Une Medecine Nouvelle; Phytotherapy et Aromatherapie. Preses de La Renaissance, Paris, 1979.

Valnet, Jean.
The Practice of Aromatherapy. Destiny Books, 1980.

Wildwood, Christine.
Aromatherapy and Massage Book. National Book, 1995.
Encyclopedia of Aromatherapy. Inner Traditions, 1996.

Worwood, Valerie Ann.
The Complete Book of Essential Oils and Aromatherapy. Pan Books, 1987.
Aromatherapy for the Healthy Child. New World Library, 2000.

Herbs, Beauty and Perfume

Busch, Julia.
Home Guide to Natural Beauty Care. Berkeley Publishing Group, 1995.

Leigh, Michelle Domonique.
Inner Peace, Outer Beauty. Carol Publishing Group, 1995.

Gladstar, Rosemary.
Herbal Healing for Women. Simon & Schuster, 1993.

Gumbel, Dietrich.
Principles of Holistic Skin Therapy with Herbal Essences. Karl F. Haug Publishers, 1986.

Hoffman, David.
The Holistic Herbal. Findhorn Press, 1983.

Maple, Eric.
The Magic of Perfume: Aromatics and Their Esoteric Significance. Samuel Weiser, 1973.

Miller, Richard and Iona.
The Magical and Ritual Use of Perfumes. Destiny Books, 1990.

Rechelbacher, Horst.
Rejuvenation: A Wellness Guide for Women and Men. Thorsons, 1987.

Rose, Jeanne.
Kitchen Cosmetics. North Atlantic Books, 1998.
Jeanne Rose's Modern Herbal. Grosset & Dunlap, 1987.

Tenny, Louise.
Today's Herbal Health. Woodland, 1997.

Van Toller, S., and Dodd, G.H.
Perfumery. The Psychology and Biology of Fragrance. Chapman & Hall, 1988.
Fragrance. The Psychology and Biology of Perfume. Elsevier Applied Science, 1992.

Minerals, Gems and Crystals

Baer, Randall and Vicki.
Windows of Light. Harper & Row, 1984.
The Crystal Connection. Harper & Row, 1987.

Bhattacharya, A.
Gemtherapy. Firma KLM Private LTD., (Calcutta) 1976.

Calverly, R.
The Language of Crystals. Radionics Research Association, 1986.

Doczi, Gyorgy
The Power of Limits, Shambhala, 1981

Gurudas.
Gem Elixirs and Vibrational Healing. Cassandra Press, 1985.

Hurlbut Jr., Cornelius, and Klein, Cornelis.
Manual of Mineralogy. John Wiley & Sons, 1977.

Hurtak, J.J.
The Book of Knowledge; The Keys of Enoch, Academy for Future Science, 1982)

Johari, Harish.
The Healing Power of Gemstones. Destiny, 1988.

Kunz, George Frederick.
The Curious Lore of Precious Stones. Dover Publications, 1913, 1971.

Melody.
Love is in the Earth. Earth Love Publishing House, 1991.
Love is in the Earth, Mineralogical Pictorial. Earth Love Publishing House, 1993.

Raphaell, Katrina.
Crystal Healing: the Therapeutic Application of Crystals and Stones. Aurora Press, 1987.

Simon & Schuster's Guide to Rocks & Minerals. Simon & Schuster, 1977.

Sofianides, Anna S. and Harlow, George E.
Gems and Crystals. Simon and Schuster, 1991.

Webster, Robert.
Gems, Their Sources, Descriptions and Identification. Butterworth & Co., 1975.

Vibrational Healing, Color, Sound and Other Related Topics:

Ardell, D.
High Level Wellness: An Alternative to Doctors, Drugs and Disease. Bantam Books, 1977, 1979.

Babbit, E.S.
The Principles of Light and Color. Citadel Press, 1967.

Becker, R., and Selden, G.
The Body Electric: Electromagnetism and the Foundation of Life. William Morrow & Co., Inc., 1985.

Brennan, Barbara Ann.
Hands of Light. Bantam, 1989.

Brodie, Renee.
The Healing Tones of Crystal Bowls. Aroma Art Ltd., 1996.

Chopra, Deepak, M.D.
Quantum Healing. Bantam, 1989.

Clark, L.
The Ancient Art of Color Therapy. Pocket Books, 1975.

David, W.
The Harmonics of Sound, Color and Vibration: A System for Self Awareness and Soul Evolution. DeVorss & Co., 1980.

Garfield, Leah Maggie.
Sound Medicine. Celestial Arts, 1987.

Gerber, Richard.
Vibrational Medicine. Bear & Company, 1988.

Gimbel, T.
Healing Through Color. Daniel, 1980.

Hunt, Roland.
The Seven Keys to Color Healing. Harper & Row, 1971.

Leadbeater, C.W.
The Chakras. Theosophical Publishing House, 1977.

Liberman, Jacob.
Light: Medicine of the Future. Bear & Company, 1993.

MacIvor, V., and LaForest, S.
Vibrations: Healing Through Color, Homeopathy and Radionics. Samuel Weiser, Inc., 1979.

Myss, Carolyn
Anatomy of a Spirit. Random House, 1997.

Oldfield, H., and Coghill, R.
The Dark Side of the Brain. Element, 1988.

Ouseley, S.G.J.
The Power of the Rays. L.N. Fowler & Co., 1986.

Powell, A.E.
The Etheric Double: The Health Aura of Man. Theosophical Publishing House, 1969.

Siegel, B.
Love, Medicine and Miracles. Harper & Row, 1986.

Summer Rain, Mary.
Earthway: A Native American Visionary Path to Total Mind, Body and Spirit Health. Pocket Book, 1992.

Tiller, W.
"Some Energy Field Observations of Man and Nature." *Kirlian Aura: Photographing the Galaxies of Life*. Doubleday, 1974.

Tompkins, Peter, and Bird, Christopher.
The Secret Life of Plants. Harper & Row, 1973.

Reputable and Organic Essential Oils Distributors:

Eden Botanicals
P.O. Box 150
Hyampom, CA 96046
888 568 9919
www.edenbotanicals.com

Original Swiss Aromatics
P.O. Box 6842
San Rafael, CA 94903
415 459 3998
www.originalswissaromatics.com

Prima Fleur
1525 E. Francisco Blvd Suite 16
San Rafael, CA 94901
415 455 0957
www.primafleur.com

PrimaVera Life
www.primavera life.com
www.goddessofspring.com

Aromatherapy Education

Aromatherapy Conference Tours
3734 131st Ave. N Suite 2
Clearwater, FL 33762
800 822 9698
aromatherapytours@verizon.net
www.aromatherapyconferencetours.com

Australasian College of Health Sciences
5940 SW Hood Ave.
Portland, Oregon 97239
800 487 8839
www.herbed.com

The Atlantic Institute of Aromatherapy
16018 Saddlestring Drive
Tampa, Florida 33612
813 265 2222
www.atlanticinstitute.com

The Northwest College for Herbal and Aromatic Studies
335 Amber Lane
Willow Spring, NC 27592
919 894 7230
www.theida.com

Michael Scholes School of Aromatic Studies
correspondence course: www.labofflowers.com

Pacific Institute of Aromatherapy
P.O. Box 6723
San Rafael, CA 94903
415 479 9120
www.pacificinstituteofaromatherapy.com

Shirley Price International College of Aromatherapy
Essentia House, Upper Bond Street
Hinckley, Leicestershire
LE10 1 RS United Kingdom
Tel: (44) 1455 615466
www.shirleyprice.co.uk

Consulting, Formulation Development, Aromatherapy Perfumery, Rare Essential Oil Sources.

EM Studios Arome
Eva-Marie Lind
Scent design
www.evamarielind.com

Esscént
Kendra Grace
Custom therapeutic perfume design, clinical
psycho-aromatherapy sessions.
P.O. Box 656
Laguna Beach, CA 92652
kendra@aromajewels.com

Lifetree Aromatix
John Steele
Exotic essential oils and hydrolates, perfume design.
3949 Longridge Ave.
Sherman Oaks, CA 91423
818 986 0594

Santa Fe Fragrance
Christine Malcolm
Fine Fragrances, manufacturing, private label, essential oils.
P.O. Box 282
Santa Fe, New Mexico 87504
505 474 0302
www.santafefragrance.com

Other Suggested Websites:

Aromajewels:
Crystals and gems, aromatic jewelry
www.aromajewels.com

Crystal bowls:
www.crystalbowls.com

Herbs:
www.mountainroseherbs.com
www.soothingherbals.com

Marcel Vogel:
www.vogelcrystals.net

Watsu:
www.waba.edu

INDEX

ABOUT THE AUTHOR

Brazilian-born Kendra Grace is one of the pioneers of classic aromatherapy in the United States. Kendra has traveled the world for over twenty years, extensively studying and researching her multifaceted background of aromatherapy, natural stones and the healing arts. She wrote the *Aromatherapy Pocketbook*, which was released in two editions, 1994 and 1999. Her writings on aromatherapy are also available in Spanish and Portuguese.

Kendra has produced, filmed and directed *Precious Essence*, a feature documentary on the distillation and history of precious flower oils, filmed on location in five continents around the world.

She invented a synergistic line of jewelry known worldwide as Aromajewels®, combining gemstones and crystals with essential oil perfumes to be used aesthetically as well as in vibrational healing.

Kendra lives with her husband and her daughter Natasha, between Laguna Beach, California and Bahia, Brazil.

To learn more about Kendra's work and buy her products visit: http://www.aromajewels.com